relieve
stress

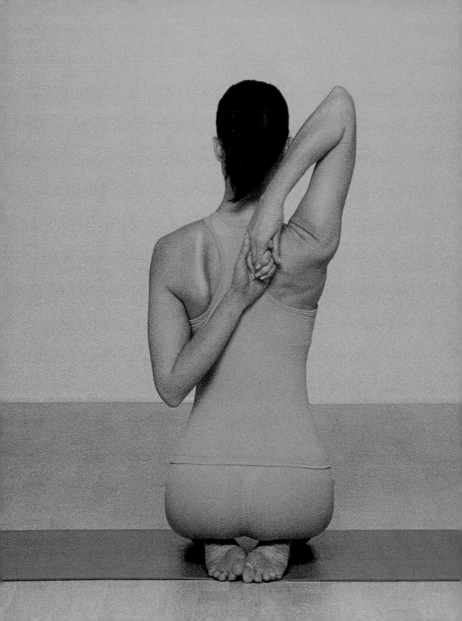

relieve
stress

Ruth Gilmore

YOGA BIOMEDICAL TRUST

A Dorling Kindersley Book

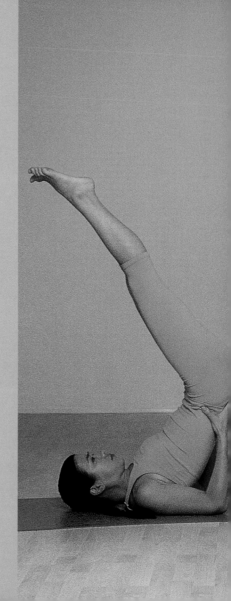

London, New York, Munich,
Melbourne, and Delhi

Series art editor: Anne-Marie Bulat
Series editor: Jane Laing

Series consultant: Peter Falloon-Goodhew
Managing editor: Gillian Roberts
Senior art editor: Karen Sawyer
Category publisher: Mary-Clare Jerram

DTP designer: Sonia Charbonnier
Production controller: Joanna Bull

Photographer: Graham Atkins-Hughes
(represented by A & R Associates)

First published in Great Britain in 2002
by Dorling Kindersley Limited,
80 Strand, London WC2R 0RL
A Penguin Company

2 4 6 8 10 9 7 5 3 1

A CIP catalogue record for this book
is available from The British Library

ISBN: 0-7513-3702-1

Colour reproduced by
Colourscan, Singapore
Printed and bound by
South China Printing Co., Hong Kong / China

See our complete catalogue at www.dk.com

contents

introduction

The appeal of yoga is universal and timeless. Its holistic practices allow you to reconnect with your real self and develop an inner calm and balance that enable you to manage stress effectively.

Your body can tolerate enormous variation in living conditions, including extremes of temperature, humidity, and altitude. It is made up of millions of cells, organized into complex organs and systems, which cooperate with one another to provide a stable internal environment in which the cells can survive, whatever is going on in the outside world.

Throughout life, the body continually responds to events and activities as required. Whether you are asleep, exercising, or even standing on your head, the body will adjust your heart rate, blood pressure, and breathing to maintain this all-important internal stability.

Any factor that threatens to overwhelm or destabilize this balance is called a stressor, and the resulting effect on the body is known as stress. Stressors can affect the body in different ways. Physical stressors

HEALTH CONCERNS

If a health practitioner has advised you not to over-exert yourself physically, or if you have any other health concerns, seek advice from a qualified yoga therapist or teacher (see p.128) before using this book. Page 17 provides basic advice for some common medical conditions and, where appropriate, "Take Care" advice or Alternatives are given for individual practices. If you are pregnant, or have recently given birth, ask a suitably qualified yoga teacher which practices would be appropriate for you.

include extremes of climate and altitude, bodily injury, exercise, and lack of sleep. Psychological factors, such as fear, grief, and anxiety, also activate the stress response.

Positive stressors

Not all stressors are detrimental to the body. We need a certain amount of stimulation to stay healthy and active. Children who are deprived of play with others and receive little or no cuddling often become adults with physical, behavioural, and psychological problems. Stressors provide stimulus, without which our minds and bodies would sink into inertia and depression.

The right amount of stress can actually enhance performance. Most public performers recognize the benefit of just enough "stage nerves", and sports people know the importance of the "adrenaline rush" in enabling them to compete to the best of their ability.

Enjoyable events and activities may also trigger stress responses. Research has shown that getting married or going on holiday can be almost as stressful as losing your job or moving house.

For optimum, all-round health you need to experience the right amount of the right types of stressors. In addition, you need to know how to cope with stressor overload or with exposure to unpleasant stressors.

Acute and chronic stress

Stress can be acute or chronic. Our bodies are designed to be able to deal with an acutely stressful situation by activating the "fright, fight, or flight" ("FFF") reaction. FFF is a reflex multi-system response produced by the sympathetic part of the nervous system. It prepares the body for the possible need either to fight or run away from danger.

The rate and depth of breathing increases. The heart rate rises, while the heart pumps more strongly. Blood is quickly redirected to the brain and muscles, and away from areas such as the skin and digestive tract, where normal function can be safely suspended during the emergency. The pupils dilate to be able to see better, and the whole body is put on a state of alert by the outpouring of the hormone adrenaline from the adrenal glands into the circulation. Adrenaline production also affects the secretion of many other hormones, coordinating the multi-system effect.

When the acute situation is over, the FFF reaction dies away. The normal state of balance is restored quite quickly, and any sense of reaction or tiredness soon disappears.

Regular exposure to too many stressors produces a more chronic state of affairs, with the FFF reaction remaining partially and continuously activated. In this state, adrenaline levels in the blood are higher than normal, and the individual feels constantly on edge, gradually less and less able to cope, and more and more exhausted.

Negative stressors

Stressors can affect the body, the mind, and the spirit. The body is put under stress if you live in a harsh environment, with marked swings of temperature and humidity, or at high altitude. Fortunately, most of us do not have this problem.

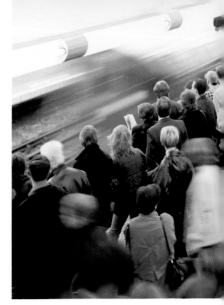

Facing the rush-hour crush morning and evening every weekday can increase your physical stress levels considerably.

Many of us do regularly experience less extreme physical stressors, such as exposure to city air pollution and environmental toxins. Uncomfortable working conditions, such as poorly designed seating or working night shifts, also affect significant numbers of people, as does crowded and unreliable public transport.

Mental stresses are more common than physical ones. Today's high-tech communication systems have contributed to the development of a faster pace of life than humankind has experienced in its entire history. Leisure time – "time for me" – can be almost impossible to find, and when a break does present itself, you may find that you have become unable to switch off and relax.

The experience of chronic stress can lead over time to a sense of dis-spiritedness. It is easy nowadays to feel that you are on a treadmill, with no respite from the daily grind.

Being in such a situation can lead to psychological illnesses, such as anxiety and depression. The effect of high levels of stress hormones, such as adrenaline and cortisol, disrupts normal physiological functions, leaving the body vulnerable to a host of physical ailments. High blood pressure, infections, allergies, skin rashes, and digestive problems are only some of the conditions made worse by chronic overstress.

Factors affecting stress levels

Modern lifestyles certainly contribute to the build-up of chronic stress. Most people work, either as employees or in self-employment.

SIGNS OF OVERSTRESS

Chronic overstress produces numerous physical, mental, and emotional signs.

• Muscle tension in the neck and shoulders causes pain and stiffness.

• Muscle tension in the scalp and jaw results in headaches and face pain. Migraines are common, as are episodes of teeth grinding at night, nail biting, fidgeting, and foot tapping.

• The heart beats faster, the breathing becomes shallow, and you sweat.

• Digestive problems produce heartburn, irritable bowel syndrome (IBS), and bowel disturbances.

• You feel driven and under constant pressure. You suffer tiredness, anxiety, depression, continual worrying, and an overactive mind that is never still.

• Attacks of insomnia add an overlying element of physical tiredness, while the inability to switch off further upsets sleep patterns.

• Panic attacks may occur, stimulating the release of even more adrenaline. The appetite can become disturbed, and increased alcohol intake can lead to alcohol dependence.

• Smoking, which many use in an attempt to de-stress, only makes matters worse by saturating the body with toxins and damaging the lungs and blood vessels.

Many employees are subject to regular performance scrutiny, with deadlines and sales targets to achieve. Salaries may contain a bonus element that can be acquired only through extra working hours. For those in management, added responsibilities increase the pressure.

Many people, especially women, are "multi-tasking", juggling careers with home and family responsibilities in addition to work commitments. This can require an almost super-human ability to plan, prioritize, and carry out numerous tasks, usually several at once. No wonder many women feel that during the years spent raising their families they are always tired, and always cross!

Lifestyle events can produce unbearable stressors. Events such as bereavement, divorce, moving house, having a baby, and changing jobs each result in considerable stress. If more than one of these significant events occurs within a short period, you may well become overstressed.

Many of us lead sedentary lives. Sometimes this is by choice, but often it is because we just cannot find the time to exercise. The body is designed to be used: without regular exercise it becomes stiff and weak.

Equally, too much exercise can be as stressful as too little. Exercise addiction, in which the body is pushed to its limits too often, has become some people's way of coping with stress. This may be connected with the desire to look like a celebrity role model, but it reveals a deep inner dissatisfaction. Unfortunately, the overall effect is to increase stress levels, not reduce them.

You can unwittingly increase your stress level by adopting poor standing and sitting postures. Sitting for long periods at work or in the car does not help; nor does standing and walking, carrying shopping bags, school bags, or toddlers, especially all at once. Such physical stressors can cause pain and tension in the neck, shoulders, and lower back.

Your mental or emotional state can affect your stress levels markedly. When faced with forthcoming examinations or an interview, you can put so much pressure on yourself to do well that you overstress yourself.

Medical conditions, especially those causing pain or chronic discomfort, increase stress levels in the sufferer. Arthritis, ME, fibromyalgia, irritable bowel syndrome, and similar conditions can make the everyday tasks of life more difficult to perform, adding to the pressure.

Modern global communications mean that most people become aware of natural and man-made disasters almost as soon as they happen, even when they are thousands of miles away. Graphic images and heart-rending interviews act as marked stressors, especially when you feel powerless to do anything.

Restoring the balance

When you are being bombarded by numerous stressors, you must review your lifestyle and determine to change it where necessary. However, before you can change the way you live, you must become aware of how you actually feel. Stress can mask the information being sent to the brain by the thousands of sensory nerve endings situated all over the body. In this way, you progressively lose touch with yourself. Consequently, you do not notice tiredness until it becomes exhaustion, or muscle tension until it becomes unbearable.

When you reach this point, it is imperative that you learn how to slow down, to get back in touch with the natural rhythms of the body,

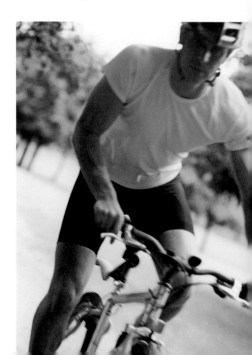

Incorporating regular exercise, such as cycling, into your routine helps keep your body fit and more able to deal with stress.

mind, and spirit. By learning to observe the body objectively you can become truly aware of how you feel, and more able to understand what is happening at times of stress.

When you are able to really get in touch with yourself, the symptoms of stress begin to reduce. Panic attacks, and other manifestations of stress, subside and you feel that they are no longer controlling you.

How can yoga help?

Yoga is the age-old lifestyle system that reconnects you with your real self. It then maintains that sensitive awareness of how things actually are, and what you really want out of life. Yoga works at all levels of the individual – through the body, mind, and spirit simultaneously.

Gentle, enjoyable stretches and asanas (traditional yoga postures) ease out muscle tensions and limber the joints, while at the same time maintaining the general health of the

body. Relaxation techniques further help the body to let go of tension and become re-energized.

In yoga, working with the breath is an integral part of the practice – the breath acts as a link between the body and the mind. Simple breathing practices encourage quietness of mind, and teach the "thinking" parts of the mind to relax and rest. These

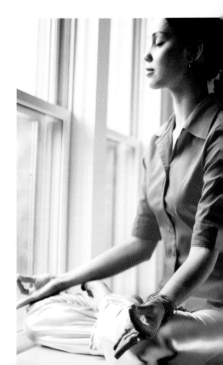

Simple breathing practices, using a mudra (symbolic hand gesture), can help you to centre yourself, restoring peace of mind and inner calm during stressful situations.

practices lead to the development of simple meditation, which deepens the experience of inner calm. This sense of tranquillity and balance is then carried into everyday life to enable you to manage and do well in the most stressful situations.

Unlike most other aspects of life, yoga is non-competitive; you work with yourself as you are. Regular practice develops self-acceptance, which in turn leads to personal growth. Many other stress-relieving practices, such as reflexology and massage, although valuable, require someone else to provide the service; with yoga, you take responsibility for yourself and your practice.

As you become accustomed to regular yoga practice you will find that you begin to live yoga on a daily basis. Your whole attitude to life changes; you no longer find yourself exasperated by the habits or actions of colleagues or family members. You are able to stay calm when events do not work out as you hoped, and you are much more able to cope with day-to-day problems and find satisfactory solutions.

HOW TO USE THIS BOOK

The rest of this book is divided into three sections. The **Foundations** section provides guidance on practising yoga and some basic breathing and preliminary stretches. Familiarize yourself with these first before moving on to the **Building Blocks** section. This contains a selection of postures and breathing practices, as well as a simple meditation and relaxation technique. Work through these postures gradually, selecting one or two to work on at a time, rather than trying to do them all in one go. Look at the photographs first to get a feel for the shape of the posture. Then follow the accompanying step-by-step instructions. If you find a posture difficult, work on the preliminary steps first or try the alternative, if one is given.

The **Programmes** section combines selected postures and other practices in a series of short yoga programmes designed for particular situations and needs. Make sure that you understand how to do the postures first before trying these programmes.

Yoga is traditionally learnt from a teacher, and you will benefit from going to a class, if you are not already doing so. Organizations that can help you find a qualified teacher in the UK are listed on page 128.

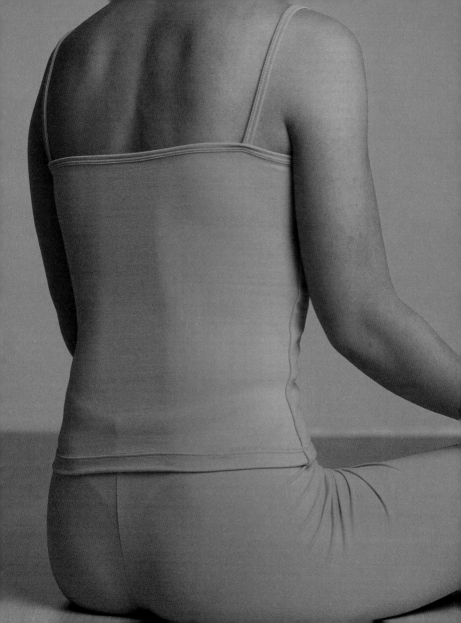

foundations

This section shows you some basic standing, sitting, and lying postures. It provides breath-with-movement exercises to loosen your body and help you deepen the connection with the breath. Breathing and centring practices are given to bring awareness to your practice.

before
you start

Yoga helps you manage stress more effectively by teaching you how to slow down and let go. Practise the postures slowly, with awareness, so that your movements are deliberate and mindful.

Try to make a particular "time for me" every day to practise yoga. A few minutes every day is better than a whole hour once or twice a week.

Always practise on an empty stomach. Allow three hours to elapse after a large meal, two hours after a light meal, and one hour after a snack, before starting your yoga practice. Wear comfortable clothes that do not restrict your movement or breathing. Practise on a mat or other non-slip surface and make sure you have sufficient space around you to extend.

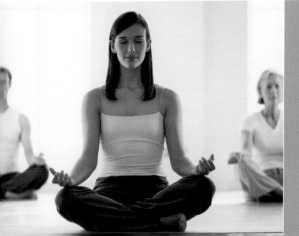

JOINING A YOGA CLASS

Practising yoga regularly in a class with the expert guidance of an experienced yoga teacher can be invaluable in helping you to manage your stress in a positive manner. Making such a commitment can help you develop your skills and abilities, and enhance the quality of relaxation and ease, reducing stress.

Act "kindly" towards yourself as you practise. Looking after yourself is very important. Never push the body into discomfort or strain, as this is counter-productive. To begin with, you may feel some stiffness for a day or two, but this will soon pass.

Support from a teacher

When you are learning to manage stress, you will find it easier if you make a commitment to attend a regular suitable yoga class. You will need to enquire in your local area to find the right sort of class for you. Organizations that can help are listed on p.128. There are many different styles available. Some emphasize physical movement and postures; some are more meditative in type.

It is hard to overestimate the value of expert guidance from a qualified yoga teacher. You may want to take up the option of beginning with some individual classes with a qualified yoga therapist before you join a general class. If you want to begin to practise at home between classes, your teacher will be able to advise you what to do.

ADVICE FOR COMMON MEDICAL CONDITIONS

• If you have high blood pressure (HBP), a heart condition, glaucoma, or detached retina, do not let your head stay below your heart.
• If you have HBP or a heart condition, hold strong standing and prone postures for a short time only. In addition, for HBP, keep your arms below your head.
• If you have low blood pressure (LBP), come up slowly from inverted poses.
• If you have a back problem or sciatica, avoid bending and twisting movements that provoke pain or other symptoms (for example, tingling or numbness in the leg). Keep your knees bent in forward bends.
• If you have a hernia, or have had recent abdominal surgery, do not put strong pressure on the abdomen.
• If you have arthritis, mobilize joints to their maximum pain-free range, but rest them if they are inflamed.
• If you have arthritis of the neck or other neck problems, do not tilt the head back in back bends and be cautious with sideways and twisting neck movements.
• During menstruation you may need to practise more gently. Avoid inversions (except for Legs up the Wall, p.70) and postures that put strong pressure on the pelvic area.

the basics

In yoga, basic standing, sitting, and lying down positions are important in their own right, helping you to develop stability and awareness of the benefits of alignment for your posture, your breathing, and for the free flow of energy. They also provide the foundations from which other postures are developed.

In addition, being able to sit comfortably and steadily is important for breathing practices and also for meditation, helping you to remain focused without distractions from physical tensions. Lying down is often used to develop body and breath awareness and to relax and allow your body to absorb the beneficial effects of other yoga practices.

If you find it impossible to achieve the full posture, it can be very helpful to use a prop, such as a block or cushion, to ensure that you do not strain your body.

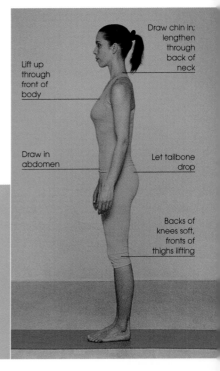

Draw chin in; lengthen through back of neck

Lift up through front of body

Draw in abdomen

Let tailbone drop

Backs of knees soft, fronts of thighs lifting

STANDING

Stand up straight with your feet parallel, hip-width apart, and your ears, tops of shoulders, hips, and ankles in line. Press your feet into the ground and lift upwards through your body. Broaden across the top of the chest. Feel balanced in every direction, as if your head is suspended by a thread from the ceiling. Look straight ahead, relax, and breathe easily.

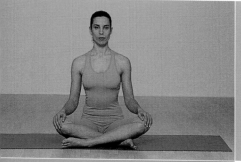

SITTING CROSS-LEGGED

This posture is good for breathing practices. Cross your shins with the feet under the opposite knee. Position yourself on the front edge of your sitting bones, with the spine long and the head erect. Relax the shoulders. If your knees are higher than your hips, sit on a block.

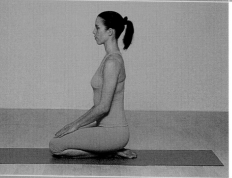

KNEELING

If you find cross-legged sitting uncomfortable, try kneeling. Sit on your heels with the tops of your thighs facing the ceiling. Or position your knees and feet hip-width apart and sit on blocks, a folded blanket, or a bolster. Keep your spine long and the head erect, the shoulders and neck relaxed.

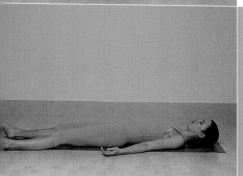

LYING ON BACK

Lie with your legs stretched out, hip-width apart. Relax the legs, and allow the feet and legs to roll outwards. Place your arms away from the body, the backs of the hands on the floor. Relax the neck and rest the centre of the back of the head on the floor.

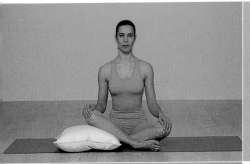

USING A CUSHION

Cushions can be used to support different parts of the body. Here one is shown supporting the thigh while sitting cross-legged. This allows the inner and the outer thigh muscles to relax, the hips to open further, and the student to stay in the posture longer without being distracted by discomfort.

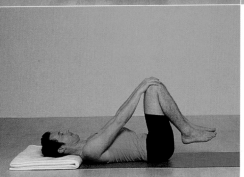

USING A BLANKET

When lying supine, the back of the neck should be long, with the chin a little down towards the chest, and not pointing up to the ceiling. If you find it difficult to keep the neck long, place a folded blanket under the head and neck for additional support.

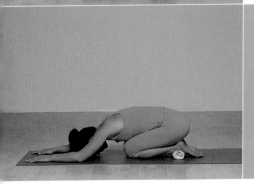

USING A TOWEL

Kneeling positions can put strain on stiff ankles. To relieve this, roll up a towel firmly and place it between the ankles and the floor. A folded towel can also be used under bony parts of the feet or ankles, especially if you are working on a hard floor.

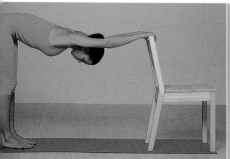

USING A CHAIR

Chairs can be used to modify postures. Shown here is a version of the Forward Bend. You can also use a chair for breathing or meditation practices if sitting or kneeling on the floor is uncomfortable. Sit towards the front of the chair, with the soles of the feet flat on the floor, hands on thighs.

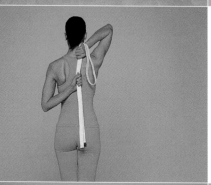

USING A BELT

A non-stretchy webbing belt or luggage strap can help you to release a stiff neck or tight shoulders. Looping a belt around the feet in some sitting postures, such as forward bends, can also help you to lift the breastbone and lengthen the spine while keeping the shoulders relaxed.

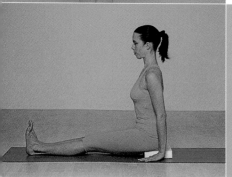

USING A FOAM BLOCK

A firm foam block will help if you find it difficult to lengthen the spine in sitting postures, as it optimizes the tilt of the pelvis. Sit towards the front of the block, not in the middle of it. If you do not have a block, use a telephone directory or small, firm cushion.

centring

Learning how to be centred is a fundamental aspect of yoga practice. It enables you to connect with your breath, becoming refreshed and re-energized from the quietness that lies within you.

In everyday life your attention is turned outwards, as you relate to the people and events around you. This can result in your energy being sapped, leaving you feeling tired and tense. The practice of centring enables you to balance your daily life with periods of quiet. You can practise centring lying on your back, sitting, or standing. Find somewhere quiet where you will not be disturbed, and make yourself comfortable.

becoming centred

1 If you choose to lie down, lie on your back, let your legs and feet roll outwards, and position your arms slightly away from your body. Keep the back of the neck long, drawing the chin gently down towards the chest. If you prefer to sit cross-legged or to stand, lift the breastbone a little and relax the shoulders.

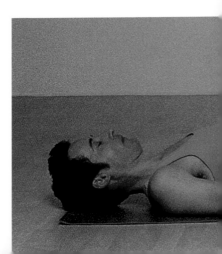

2 Close the eyes gently. Relax the scalp. Relax the face and release any tension in the jaw. Turn your attention inward, and get in touch with your body and how it feels. Begin to notice the gentle movement of the body with the breath. Feel the sensations within your body that result from these movements.

3 Be aware that you are not making the breath happen; neither are you controlling it in any way. Rather, you are trusting the body to breathe just as you do while you are asleep. Let your breath settle into a slow, deep, natural rhythm. Observe it flowing in and out of your body.

4 Let your attention be with your breath and the sensations in the body for a little while. You will find even a few breaths like this helpful, or you can practise for several minutes.

5 When you notice that your attention has wandered and you are thinking of something else, gently draw your awareness back to your breath, without analysis or judgment. It does not matter if your thoughts stray often at first. All you have to do is to keep bringing your attention back to the breath each time that it happens. The mind soon gets used to focusing lightly on the breath without strain. All it takes is a little practice.

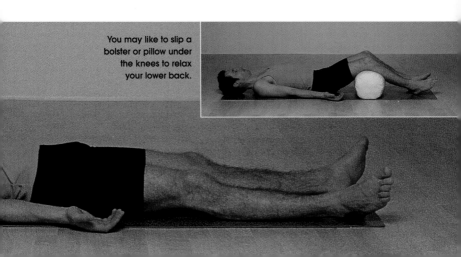

You may like to slip a bolster or pillow under the knees to relax your lower back.

basic breathing

There is a fundamental connection between the breath and your physical, mental, and emotional states. By working with the breath, you will be able to let go of stress in any situation.

Breathing provides oxygen for the metabolic processes from which we derive the energy to move, think, and feel, and carries away carbon dioxide, the main waste product of our metabolism. Physical tension in the respiratory muscles between and within the ribs can cause tightness in the chest, and even chest pain. Relaxed breathing techniques will release tension from the whole of the upper body, including the neck and shoulders. This will improve your ability to adjust your breathing to meet changing requirements.

The breath also provides a powerful link between mind and body. By controlling your breathing patterns – for example, the rhythm and depth of breathing, the length of the out-breath, and the balance between right and left nostril – you can influence your physical, mental, and emotional states.

Good breathing habits

Yoga encourages breathing through the nose, full use of the diaphragm, a slow, smooth breathing pattern, and coordination of movement and breath. Opening movements, such as back bends, are practised on an in-breath and closing movements, such as forward bends, on the out-breath.

The breathing practice opposite will help develop awareness of the action of respiratory muscles and encourage good breathing habits. It can be done standing, lying down, or sitting as well as kneeling.

sitting sectional breathing

Sectional breathing helps release muscle tension associated with poor breathing habits. After completing Step 3, combine all three steps to produce full, continuous in-breaths and out-breaths.

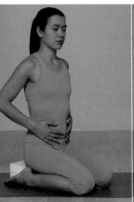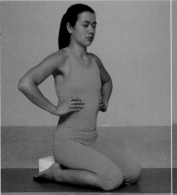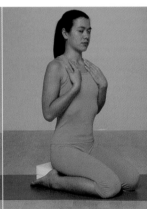

1 Kneel comfortably with your palms resting on your abdomen, the middle fingers just touching. Breathe into your hands, feeling the abdomen swell out and the fingers move apart as you breathe in. Then, feel the abdomen sink back as you exhale. Take six even breaths.

2 Bring your hands to your rib cage, with your fingers to the front and thumbs on the back ribs. Feel the ribs expand into the hands on the in-breath and relax back inwards as you exhale. Take six breaths, breathing into the sides of the chest.

3 Place your fingers on your collar bones, in front of your shoulders. Breathe in, feeling the fingers and shoulders rise up towards the head, and the top of the chest expand. As you breathe out, feel the fingers sink back down with the chest. Take six breaths.

breath with movement

These simple postures are designed to deepen your connection with your breath as well as gently moving the joints. Each movement is timed to match the length of the breath.

supine arms over head

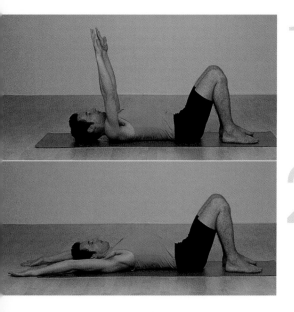

1 Lie with your knees bent and your feet on the floor. Place the feet and knees hip-width apart, arms alongside the body with the palms down. Connect with your breath. As you breathe in, bring the arms slowly and smoothly up and back behind the head.

2 Soften the elbows and relax the shoulders, so that the arms are on the floor behind your head by the time you have completed the in-breath. As you breathe out, slowly return the arms to the starting position alongside the body. Repeat for six to eight breaths.

supine nurturing

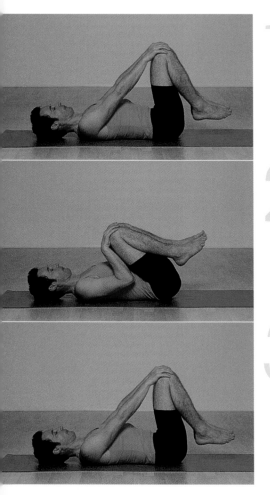

1 Lie on your back. Draw the knees up and place one hand on each kneecap, with the fingers pointing towards the feet, the knees together. Relax your shoulders. As you breathe in, send the knees away from you.

2 As you breathe out, draw the knees in towards the chest, bending your arms. Keep the shoulders relaxed and the neck long throughout.

3 As you breathe in, straighten your arms enough to send the knees away from you. Continue these movements, coordinated with the breath, for 10 to 12 breaths. This simple moving posture is one of the best for relieving stress. It also eases the back and hips when you have been sitting for long periods.

supine legs up arms out

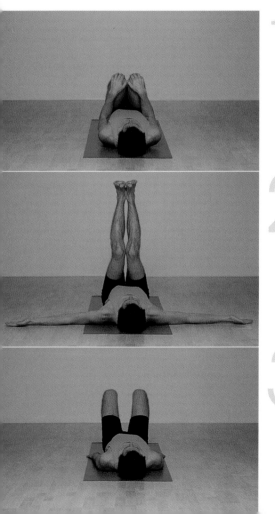

1 Lie on your back with the knees bent. Draw up the knees and place one hand over each kneecap, the fingers pointing towards the feet. Relax the shoulders and draw the chin a little down towards the chest, so that the back of the neck is long.

2 As you breathe in, take the arms out to the floor at shoulder height. At the same time, take the feet up towards the ceiling. Keep the feet together and the knees slightly bent.

3 As you breathe out, bring your legs back down slowly and place your hands on your kneecaps again. Repeat for six to eight breaths. Find a comfortable breathing rate and let your movements be governed by the breath. Then bring the feet to the floor, arms either side of the body.

supine twist

1 Lie with the knees bent, the feet together on the floor close to the hips. Position the arms away from the body at an angle of about 45 degrees. Relax the shoulders.

2 As you breathe out, slowly let the knees sink over to the left. Your hips will roll so that you are now lying more on the left hip. Turn the head to the right. Relax the feet. As you breathe in, slowly return to the starting position.

3 As you breathe out, slowly let the knees sink over to the right, turning the head to the left. Keep the shoulders and feet relaxed. As you breathe in, slowly return to the starting position. Repeat the sequence for six to eight breaths. Feel the quietening effects as you work with the breath.

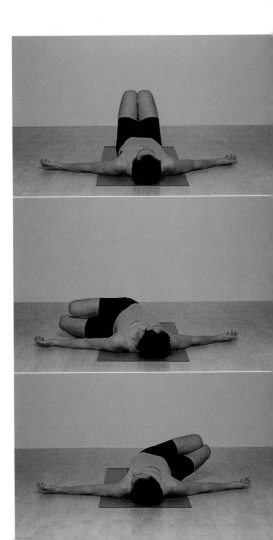

standing arm stretches

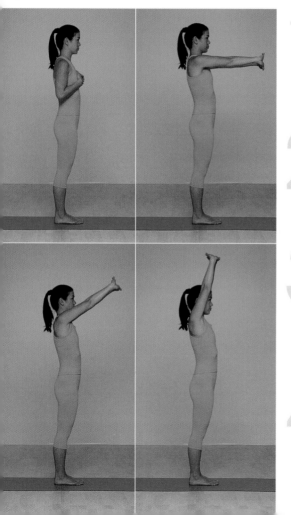

1 Stand, feet together. Become aware of the flow of the breath. Clasp your hands and place them over the breast bone. Keep the elbows and shoulders relaxed.

2 As you breathe in, turn the palms out and stretch them away from you, straightening the elbows. As you breathe out, return to the starting position. Repeat twice.

3 As you breathe in, turn the palms away and stretch them up away from you at an angle of 45 degrees, keeping the shoulders relaxed. As you breathe out, return to the starting position. Repeat twice.

4 As you breathe in, turn the palms away and stretch them right up vertically, keeping the shoulders relaxed. As you breathe out, return to the starting position. Repeat twice more, then unclasp the hands.

cafetière stretch

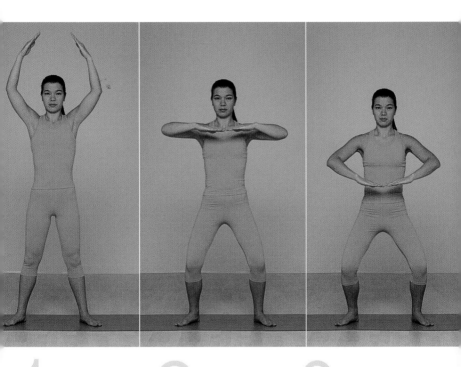

1 Stand with the feet more than hip-width apart and the toes turned out. As you breathe in, stretch the arms out to the sides, palms up, and circle them up to almost meet above your head.

2 Imagine you have in front of you a huge cafetière plunger. As you breathe out, bring your arms in front of your chest until your fingers touch. Bend slightly at the knees and begin to push down with your hands.

3 Continue to push down the imaginary plunger until your hands are level with your waist. Then repeat four to six times, coordinating the actions with the breathing.

neck stretches

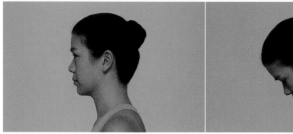

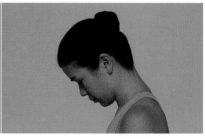

1 These gentle movements ease out muscle tension in the neck and shoulders. Sit cross-legged on the floor or on an upright chair. Lift the breastbone and relax the shoulders.

2 Allow the head to come forward slowly under its own weight, bringing the chin down towards the chest. Keep the breastbone up. Stay in this position for several breaths.

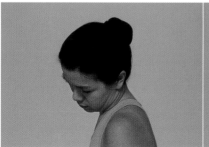

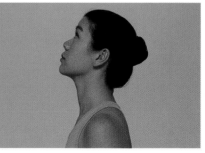

3 Allow the head to roll slowly to the left until the ear is over the shoulder. Stay for several breaths, then return to the midline position and repeat on the right. Return to the starting position.

4 Lift the chin slowly towards the ceiling, keeping the back of the neck long. Feel the stretch in all parts of the neck, hold for a few breaths, and return to the starting position.

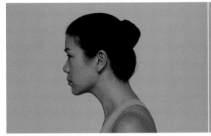

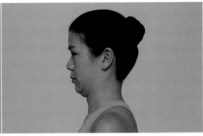

Looking forwards, slowly send the chin forward, keeping it parallel to the floor. Hold for a few breaths. Keep the shoulders relaxed throughout.

Slowly draw the chin back as far as you comfortably can, keeping it parallel to the floor. Hold for a few breaths, and then return to the starting position.

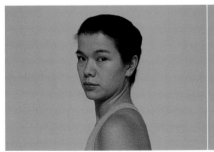

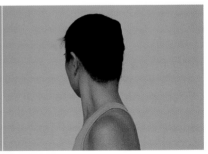

Keeping the shoulders relaxed, slowly turn the head to look over the left shoulder as far as you comfortably can. Hold for several breaths.

Return to the starting position, then turn the head to look over the right shoulder as far as you comfortably can. Hold for several breaths.

standing upward stretch

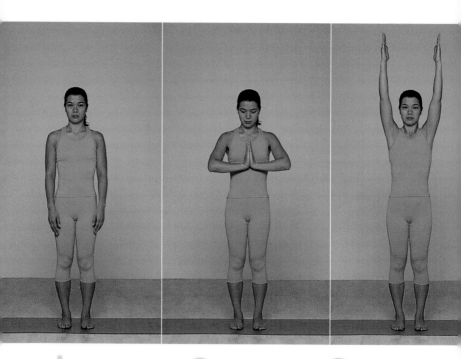

1 Stand with the feet parallel and a little apart. Rock a bit on your feet to balance your body weight evenly. Feel balanced and grounded, letting your weight pass into the floor.

2 Gently lift the kneecaps up a little, relax the shoulders, and lift up the breastbone. Bring the palms together in front of the heart. Look down at the floor past your hands.

3 Slowly stretch the arms up above your head, the palms facing one another. On an in-breath, lift up the chest and stretch. On the out-breath, bring the arms down and allow them to relax.

half forward bend

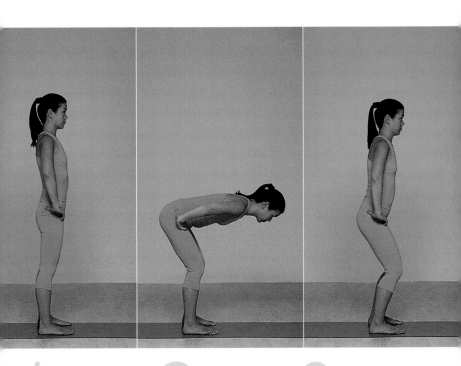

1 Stand with the feet hip-width apart, the inside edges of the feet parallel. Take your hands to the crease at the top of the leg, where the leg joins the body. Your hip joints lie behind your hands.

2 Lift the breastbone up away from the floor, to lengthen the front of the body. On an out-breath, stretch forward with a straight back until your upper body is parallel to the floor. Look down.

3 Bend the knees when you feel the stretch in the backs of the legs. Connect with your breath for several breaths. On an in-breath, come up slowly with knees bent, and return to Step 1.

standing back arch

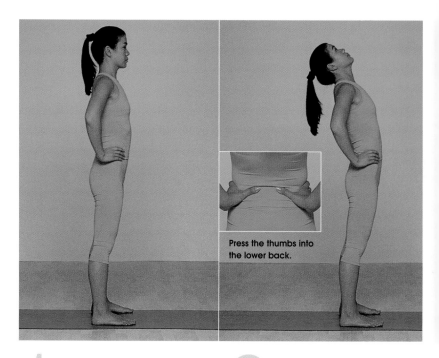

Press the thumbs into the lower back.

1 Stand with the feet hip-width apart and the inside edges of the feet parallel, the hands on the hips. Take the hands back a little, so that the thumbs rest against the lower back, several centimetres apart. Roll the shoulders back to open up the chest. Tuck the chin in.

2 Begin to lift the breastbone up away from the floor. As you lift, feel the upper body arching back. Now lift the chin to look towards the ceiling and breathe for several breaths. Keep lifting the breastbone. Slowly release the pose by lifting the breastbone as you return to an upright position.

standing side stretch

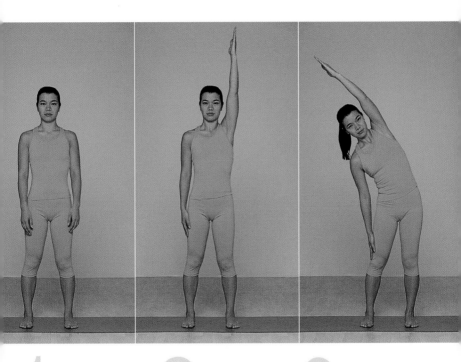

1 Stand with your feet parallel and hip-width apart, your arms down by your sides. If you have back problems, place your right hand on your hip.

2 As you breathe in, raise the left arm up beside your head, fingers reaching up to the ceiling, shoulders relaxed down away from the ears. Try to bring the raised arm to touch the left ear.

3 Reach up and out to the right on an out-breath. Hold, then return to an upright position on an in-breath. Circle the arm back down on the out-breath. Repeat on the other side.

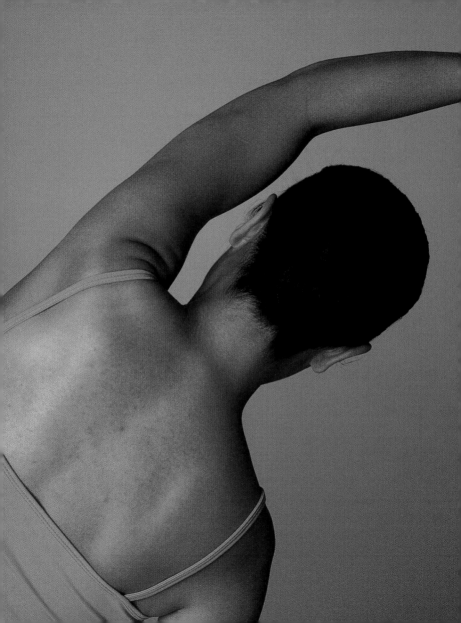

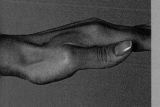

building
blocks

This section presents a variety of postures and other yoga practices to calm body, mind, and spirit. Stay in the postures only for as long as you are able to hold them steadily and comfortably, breathing evenly. Listen to your body as you practise and you will make steady progress.

eagle

This posture opens and stretches across the upper back, neck, and shoulders, releasing tension in these areas. The arms represent the eagle's folded wings and the fingers represent the feathers.

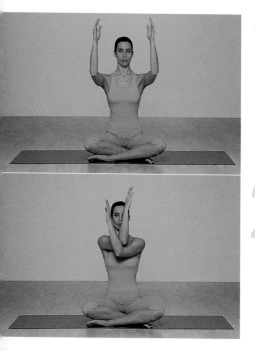

1 Sit cross-legged on the floor (use a foam block or small cushion, if necessary), hands on knees. Lift the breastbone and relax the shoulders. Bring both arms up in front of you, palms facing each other. Bend the elbows and hold them at shoulder height and shoulder-width apart, so that each arm forms a right angle.

2 Lower the left elbow a little and send the left hand away from you slightly. As you breathe in, bring the arms towards and past each other, hooking the left elbow under the right one.

TAKE CARE
• If you have neck problems, tilt the head a little forward.
• If you have stiff shoulders, do not strain to achieve the final position.

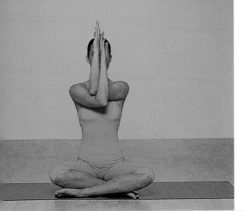

3 Breathing out, bring the backs of the forearms and the backs of the hands towards each other directly in front of your face. Bring them as close together as you can without straining your shoulders. Now let the breath flow in and out naturally.

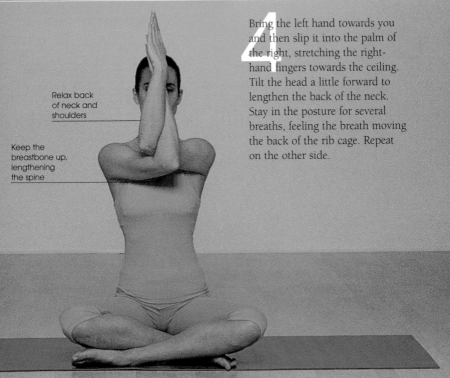

Relax back of neck and shoulders

Keep the breastbone up, lengthening the spine

4 Bring the left hand towards you and then slip it into the palm of the right, stretching the right-hand fingers towards the ceiling. Tilt the head a little forward to lengthen the back of the neck. Stay in the posture for several breaths, feeling the breath moving the back of the rib cage. Repeat on the other side.

COW

This posture stretches across the front of the body, opening the armpits and releasing tension in the neck and shoulders. As the breath is in the rib cage, the posture has an overall energizing effect.

1 Assume the basic kneeling position. Lift the breastbone and relax the shoulders. Take the left arm up the back, positioning the back of the hand between the shoulder blades, or as high as it will comfortably reach. To help position the left hand, reach behind you with the right hand and, holding on to the left elbow, draw it towards the trunk.

2 Breathing in, raise the right arm vertically. Lift the ribs on the right side of the chest, open the armpit and stretch the hand to the ceiling.

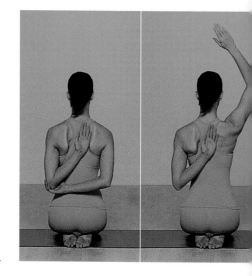

TAKE CARE
If you find one side easier than the other, practise the stiffer side before the "good" side, then repeat on the stiffer side again.

3 Bend the elbow of the right arm and lower the right hand down your back. Breathing out, hook the two hands together, then relax the neck. Hold the pose for several breaths, feeling the front of the rib cage moving with the breath. Release your hands and repeat with the left arm in the raised position.

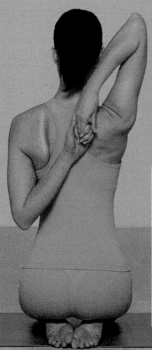

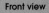

Front view

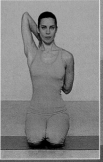

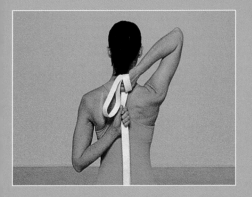

ALTERNATIVE

If the hands do not make contact, use a belt. Hold it in the right hand and lower it down behind you, reaching up for it with the left hand. When both hands are holding the belt, gather it in until the hands are comfortably close, and relax the neck.

forward
bend

Forward-stretching postures have a quietening effect on the mind. In the Forward Bend, you bend at the hips, keeping the back straight and the sitting bones lifting up to help release tight hamstrings.

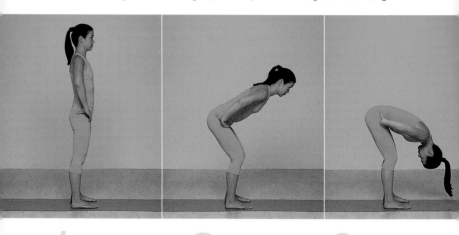

1 Stand with the feet hip-width apart and parallel. Take your hands to the crease at the tops of the legs at the point where they join the torso.

2 Lift the breastbone up away from the floor to lengthen the front of the body. As you breathe out, fold forwards from the hips, bending slightly at the knees.

3 With your knees still bent, allow the spine to relax and lengthen as gravity pulls the head and upper body down towards the floor. Breathe easily.

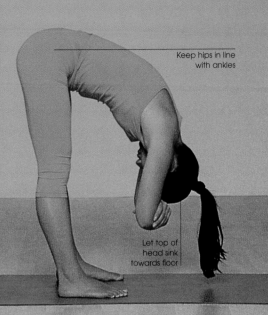

4 Letting the upper body hang from the hips, press the feet into the floor and lift your sitting bones upwards to lengthen through the backs of the legs. Bring your arms above your head, and hold on to your elbows. Stay in the position for several breaths, keeping the stretch through the backs of the legs.

Keep hips in line with ankles

Let top of head sink towards floor

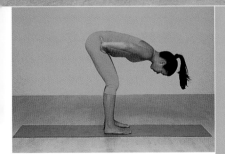

5 Bend your knees. Put your hands on your hips and come up half-way, lengthening through the upper spine. On an in-breath, come up to the basic standing position, hingeing from the hips and keeping your back straight.

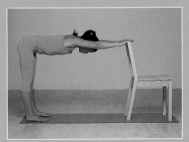

ALTERNATIVE

If you have HBP, glaucoma, or detached retina, do a Half Forward Bend, resting your hands on the back of a chair. Keep the abdomen pulled back towards the spine and the chest lifted.

tree

In Tree, not only is the body balanced, but the mind becomes quiet and relaxed, too. This posture strengthens the leg muscles and promotes good alignment of the spine.

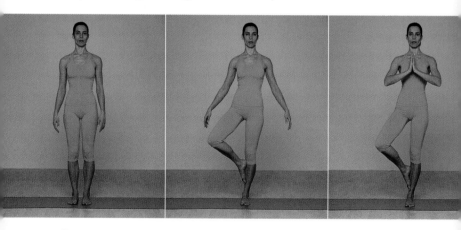

1 Stand up straight with your feet a little apart, your weight evenly distributed over both feet, and the arms by your sides.

2 Inhaling, bring the sole of the right foot against the inside of the standing leg just below the knee. Take the knee out to the side, to open the hip joint on that side.

3 As you breathe out, lift the breastbone up and relax the shoulders. Bring the palms together in front of your chest. Stop here if you have arthritis in the knees.

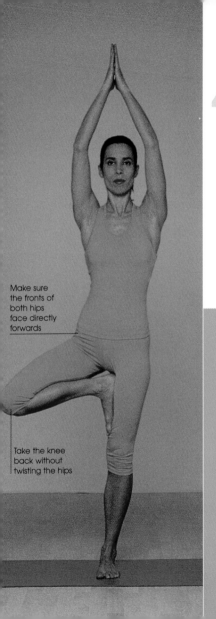

Make sure the fronts of both hips face directly forwards

Take the knee back without twisting the hips

If you feel balanced, lift the foot and place the sole against the top of the inside of the standing leg. Breathing in, stretch your arms up above the head, keeping the palms together. Relax the shoulders and the face. To stay balanced, fix your gaze on a vertical line, such as the edge of a door. Breathe easily for several breaths, then release the pose. Pause and repeat on the other side.

TAKE CARE

If bringing the palms together creates tension in the neck or shoulders, keep the hands shoulder-width apart above the head.

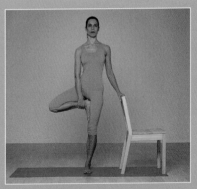

ALTERNATIVE

If your balance is poor, stand against a wall for support or hold on to the back of a chair, as shown. Holding the ankle of the raised leg may also be helpful.

side
warrior

This standing posture not only strengthens the body but also enables you to become aware of the boundless reserves of inner strength that lie within you. Stay balanced and focused throughout.

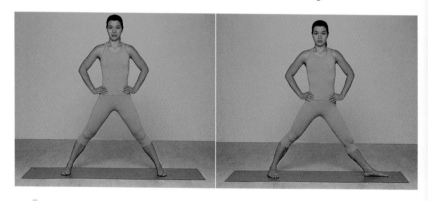

1 Stand with your feet about 1 m (3 ft) apart, the inside edges of the feet parallel, your hands on your waist and the shoulders relaxed. Look straight ahead.

2 As you breathe in, turn the toes of the right foot in a little and turn all of the left leg out from the hip 90 degrees. Keep your upper body facing front.

TAKE CARE
- If you have HBP or a heart condition, hold for a short time only.
- Proceed cautiously if you have back problems.

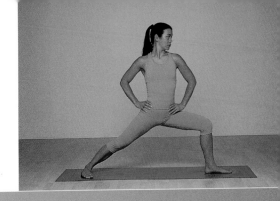

3 Breathing out, bend the left knee and allow your hips to sink towards the floor. Align the knee with the ankle to make a right angle with the leg. Turn your head to the left but keep the shoulders facing the front.

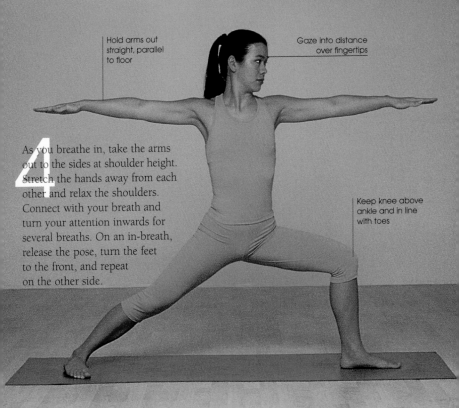

Hold arms out straight, parallel to floor

Gaze into distance over fingertips

4 As you breathe in, take the arms out to the sides at shoulder height. Stretch the hands away from each other and relax the shoulders. Connect with your breath and turn your attention inwards for several breaths. On an in-breath, release the pose, turn the feet to the front, and repeat on the other side.

Keep knee above ankle and in line with toes

lunge
warrior

Lunge warrior provides a powerful stretch through the back of the leg, thigh, and hip, extends the spine, and opens the chest. Feel the energy building as you breathe deeply into the rib cage.

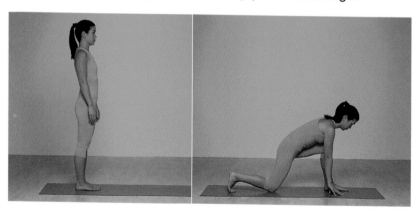

1 Stand up straight, feet hip-width apart, arms by your sides. Move on to all fours, keeping your toes curled under. Place your hands beneath the shoulders and knees beneath the hips.

2 As you exhale, take your left leg forward between your hands, so that your knee is directly above the heel of your left foot. Rest your upper body on the left thigh. Press your fingertips into the floor.

TAKE CARE
If you have back problems, do not go beyond Step 2 to begin with.

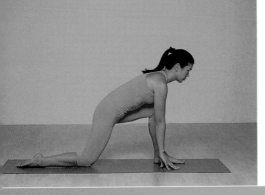

3 Keeping your fingers steepled, raise your head a little to look slightly further ahead. Untuck the toes of your right foot, so that the top of the foot is resting on the floor.

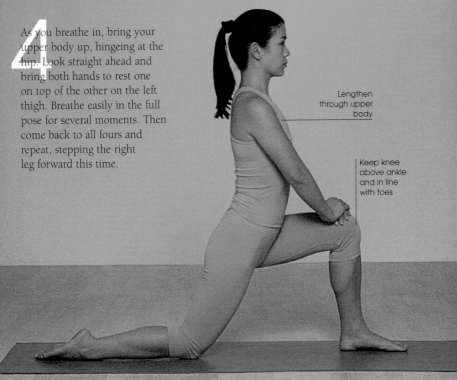

4 As you breathe in, bring your upper body up, hingeing at the hip. Look straight ahead and bring both hands to rest one on top of the other on the left thigh. Breathe easily in the full pose for several moments. Then come back to all fours and repeat, stepping the right leg forward this time.

Lengthen through upper body

Keep knee above ankle and in line with toes

downward
dog

One of the great classical yoga postures, Downward Dog works and stretches the whole body, releasing tension and quietening the mind as it balances the upper and lower body.

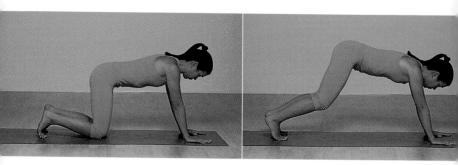

1 Begin on all fours, hands under the shoulders, feet and knees hip-width apart. Lift each hand in turn and place the heel of the hand where the fingertips were, to reposition your hands one hands-length forward, as shown. Tuck the toes under.

2 On an out-breath, come up on your toes and lift your hips up and back. Keeping your knees bent, push your hands against the floor to send your weight back towards your feet. Lengthen through the spine.

TAKE CARE
If you have back problems, keep the knees bent throughout or do the Alternative (right).

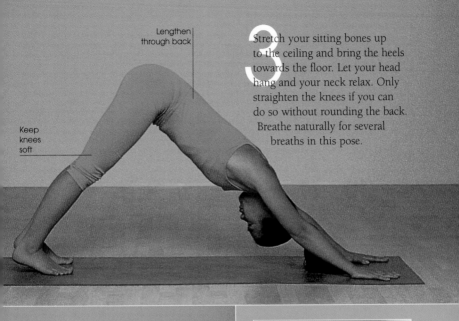

Lengthen
through back

Keep
knees
soft

3 Stretch your sitting bones up to the ceiling and bring the heels towards the floor. Let your head hang and your neck relax. Only straighten the knees if you can do so without rounding the back. Breathe naturally for several breaths in this pose.

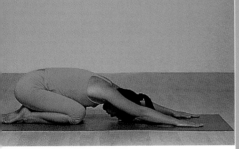

4 On an out-breath, lower the knees to the floor and, keeping your hands still, sit back on your heels in Hare (see p.81). Relax the arms and stay for a few breaths. Feel the stretch through the spine.

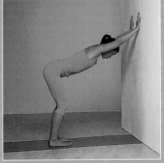

ALTERNATIVE

If you have HBP, detached retina or glaucoma, do the pose with your hands against a wall or on a chair.

cobra

Cobra extends the spine, strengthening the muscles in the back and stretching the front of the body. It also opens the chest, strengthens the diaphragm, and releases tension in the shoulders.

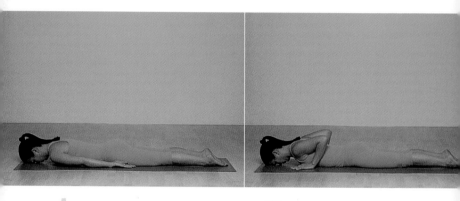

1 Lie on your front, forehead on the floor and feet hip-width apart. Let your arms lie down by your sides, palms facing upwards. Stretch the feet away along the floor.

2 Place your hands under the shoulders, spread your fingers, middle finger pointing forwards. Keep the elbows close to the body and tuck your tailbone under. Roll the shoulders back.

TAKE CARE
• Avoid if you have facet joint problems in the spine.
• If you have arthritis in the neck, keep the head in line with the spine.

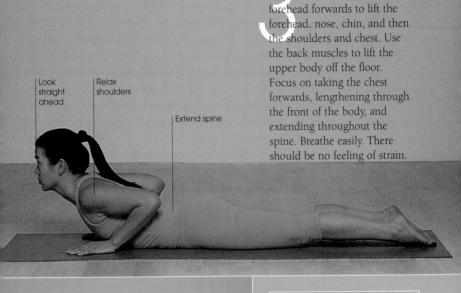

3 As you breathe in, slide the forehead forwards to lift the forehead, nose, chin, and then the shoulders and chest. Use the back muscles to lift the upper body off the floor. Focus on taking the chest forwards, lengthening through the front of the body, and extending throughout the spine. Breathe easily. There should be no feeling of strain.

Look straight ahead

Relax shoulders

Extend spine

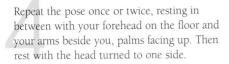

4 Repeat the pose once or twice, resting in between with your forehead on the floor and your arms beside you, palms facing up. Then rest with the head turned to one side.

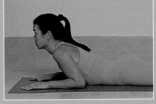

ALTERNATIVE

If you are stiff in the shoulders or have a rounded upper spine (kyphosis), you may prefer to place your hands beside your face and keep your forearms on the floor as you lift up the upper body.

locust

This back-arching posture stretches the whole body and raises the spirits. It provides a balanced strengthening of the back muscles. Practise with the breath to avoid strain and keep the mind focused.

1 Lie on your front with your forehead on the floor, the feet a little apart, and the arms by your sides. Relax completely for a few breaths.

2 Breathing out, stretch the feet away from you along the floor. Stretch the arms up and back behind you like wings. Keep your forehead pressed on the floor.

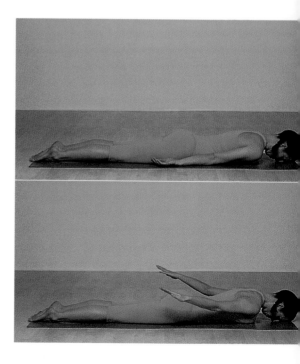

3 As you breathe in, slide the nose and chin along the floor. Lift the head and the upper body a little. Lift both legs straight up from the hip, contracting the lower back muscles. Feel the whole body lengthening. As you breathe out, slowly lower the body to the floor and relax briefly. Repeat four to six times.

Keep back of neck long

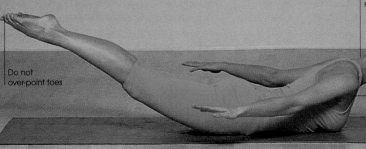

Do not over-point toes

Stretch breastbone forwards

4 On the final lowering of the body, turn the head to one side and relax the body completely. Be aware of the lower back rising and falling with the breath.

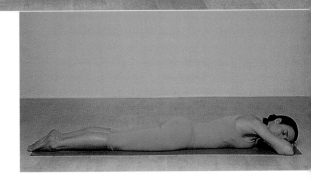

TAKE CARE
Avoid this pose if you have a peptic ulcer, hernia, or spinal facet joint problems.

half
bow

The Half Bow posture works the back, while gently stretching the front thigh and hip-flexor muscles. It is a good forerunner to the full Bow, and has an invigorating, energizing effect.

1 Lie on your front with your forehead on the floor, the feet a little apart and your arms by the sides, palms facing up.

2 As you breathe in, stretch your right arm above your head, palm facing the floor. Point the fingers away from the body. Keep resting your forehead on the floor.

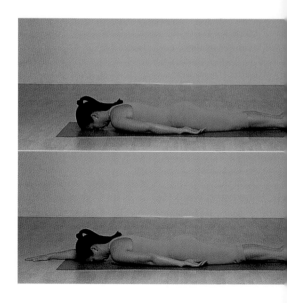

TAKE CARE
• If you have HBP, heart disese, or a hernia, do not hold final position.
• If you have back problems, stop if symptoms are provoked.

3 Exhaling, bend your left leg so that your calf touches your thigh, and take hold of the front of the ankle with your left hand. Continue to keep your forehead on the floor.

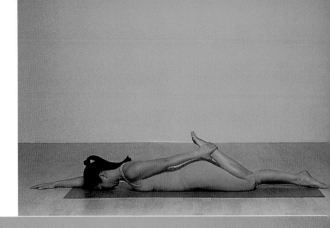

4 As you breathe in, lift the left thigh, and raise the foot away from the buttock. At the same time, lift the right arm, chest, and head together. Pause as you breathe out. Hold the position for as long as is comfortable, breathing deeply. Then, exhaling, relax the leg and lower yourself back to the floor. Repeat on the other side.

Keep arm straight

Raise thigh from floor

Look straight ahead

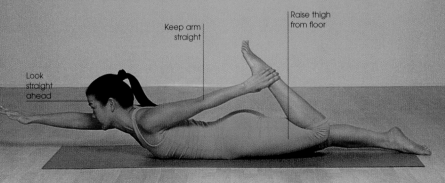

bow

Bow strengthens and tones the back and abdominal muscles, and extends the spine. It also opens the chest, stimulating deep breathing, and results in an increased sense of wellbeing.

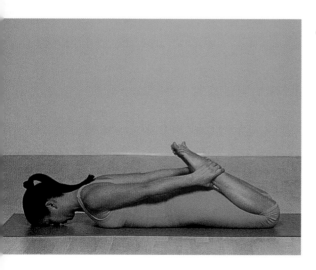

1 Lie on your front, with your legs and feet together, and your arms by your sides, palms facing up. Rest your forehead on the floor. As you breathe out, bend both legs so that the calves touch the thighs. At the same time, reach back with your arms and take hold of the fronts of the ankles.

TAKE CARE
Avoid if you have heart problems, HBP, a hernia, or back problems; start with Half Bow (see p.58).

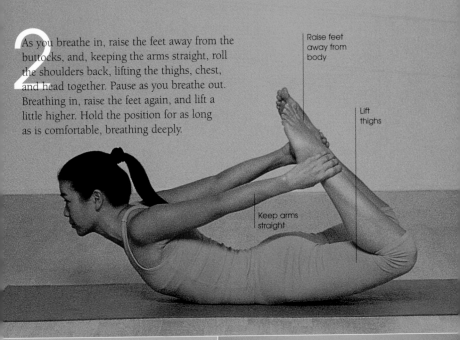

2 As you breathe in, raise the feet away from the buttocks, and, keeping the arms straight, roll the shoulders back, lifting the thighs, chest, and head together. Pause as you breathe out. Breathing in, raise the feet again, and lift a little higher. Hold the position for as long as is comfortable, breathing deeply.

Raise feet away from body

Lift thighs

Keep arms straight

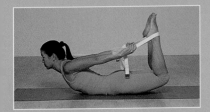

ALTERNATIVE

If you cannot reach your ankles with your hands without straining, use a belt. Wrap it around the ankles and hold the ends with both hands. Draw your chest up as you lift your thighs and raise your feet.

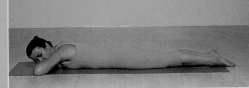

3 On an out-breath, relax the legs and lower your body to the floor. Fold your arms and rest for a few breaths with your head turned to one side, resting on the backs of your hands.

sun salute

This dynamic sequence energizes the whole body. Try to make the sequence flowing by coordinating movement with breath. After completing the sequence, repeat on the other side of the body.

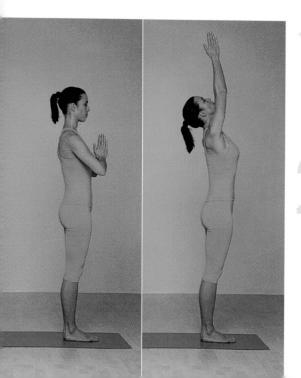

1 Stand up straight with your feet together, and your palms pressed together in prayer position in front of your chest. Look straight ahead. Centre yourself and then inhale fully.

2 As you breathe in, take your arms out to the sides of your body, turning the palms out, and lift both arms up above your head. Bring your palms together and lift up the breastbone. Open your chest as you look up at your hands. Do not let the head fall back and keep the shoulders relaxed.

3 Breathing out, fold forwards from the hips over bent legs into a relaxed Forward Bend (see p.44). Bend your arms above your head and hold at the elbows. Let the torso hang. Stay in this position for three to four breaths.

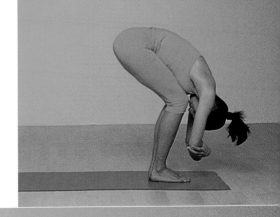

4 Exhaling, come into Lunge Warrior (see p.50). Take a large step back with your right foot, landing on the ball of the right foot. Lower the right knee to the floor and rest your upper torso on your left thigh. Steeple your fingers. Stretch the breastbone forwards and look straight ahead. Stay in the position for three to four breaths. ▶

Keep back of neck long

Knee touches floor

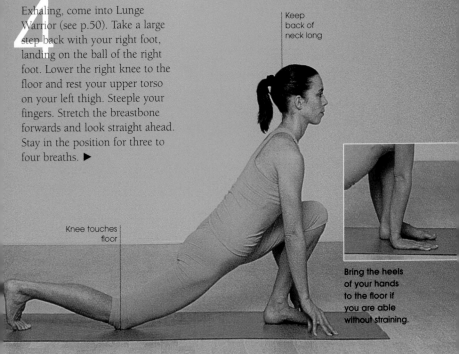

Bring the heels of your hands to the floor if you are able without straining.

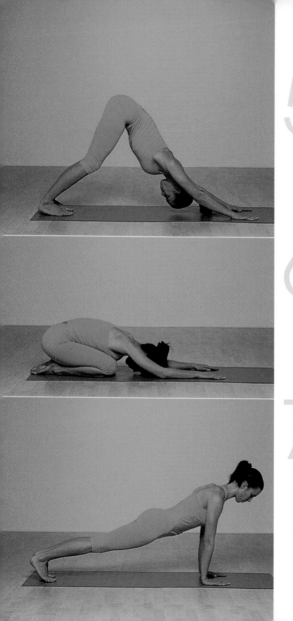

5 Exhale as you step the left foot back to come into Downward Dog (see p.52). Press your heels towards the floor and bend the knees if necessary. Do not force your heels onto the floor. Let your head hang, your neck relax. Stay in the position for three to four breaths.

6 On an out-breath, bring your knees to the floor and, keeping your hands still, move into Hare (see p.81). Rest in this pose for three to four breaths.

7 Breathing in, bring your body forward and lift your legs and torso off the floor, tucking your toes under. Your hands should be directly beneath your shoulders. Maintain a straight line with your body and legs. Look down at the floor. Hold the position and breathe out.

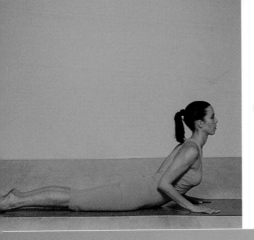

8 Breathing in, lower yourself to the floor into Cobra (see p.54). Keep the hands directly underneath the shoulders and the elbows tucked in. Focus on taking the chest forwards, lengthening through the front of the body, and extending throughout the spine.

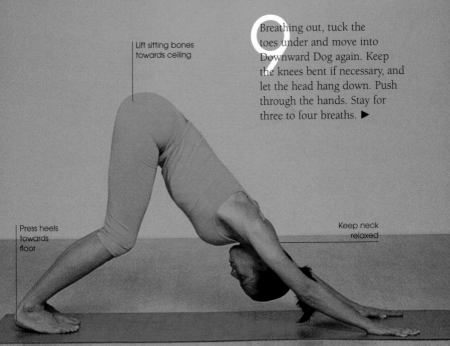

Lift sitting bones towards ceiling

Press heels towards floor

Keep neck relaxed

9 Breathing out, tuck the toes under and move into Downward Dog again. Keep the knees bent if necessary, and let the head hang down. Push through the hands. Stay for three to four breaths. ▶

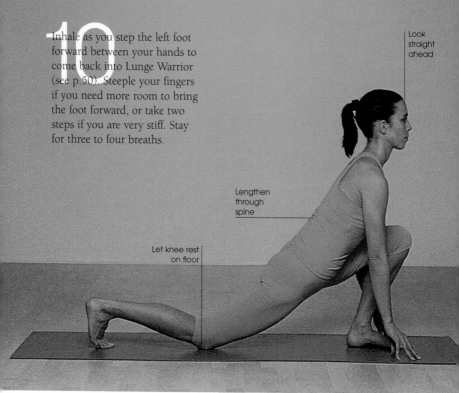

10 Inhale as you step the left foot forward between your hands to come back into Lunge Warrior (see p.50). Steeple your fingers if you need more room to bring the foot forward, or take two steps if you are very stiff. Stay for three to four breaths.

Look straight ahead

Lengthen through spine

Let knee rest on floor

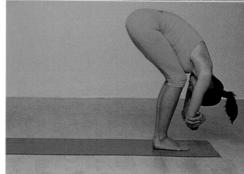

11 As you exhale, bring your right foot forward to join the left foot and come into an easy Forward Bend with bent legs (see p.44). Bend your arms above your head and hold on to the elbows. Relax in this position for three to four breaths.

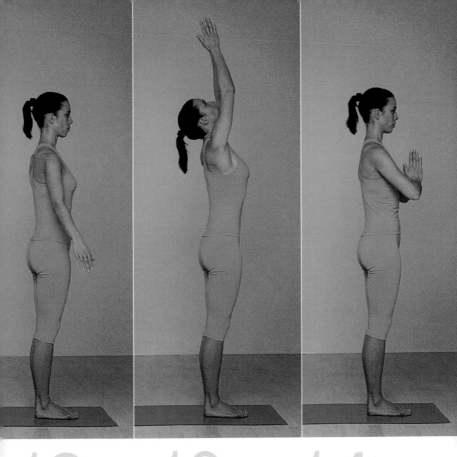

12 Breathing in, roll the body up slowly, keeping the knees bent until you are completely upright. Breathe out once when you are standing up straight.

13 Breathing in, circle your arms out to the sides and then over your head. Bring the palms together and look up at your hands. Lift the breastbone but do not bend backwards.

14 Breathing out, bring your arms down in front of your chest in prayer position. Look straight ahead and breathe easily for a few minutes. Repeat the sequence on the other side.

bridge

Bridge is a back-arching posture that also opens the chest and releases neck and shoulder tension. It is especially soothing if practised moving on the out-breath only.

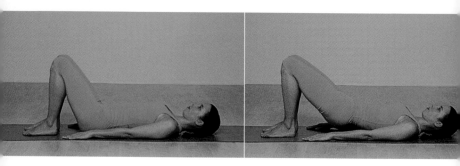

1 Lie on your back with your knees drawn up and your feet hip-width apart. Allow a hand's length of space between the hips and the heels. Have the arms alongside the body with the palms facing down. Draw the chin a little down towards the chest, to lengthen the back of the neck.

2 Breathe in, feeling the length of your back on the floor. As you breathe out, push your feet against the floor to lift the hips and then the back off the floor as far as you comfortably can. Make sure your feet are directly beneath the knees, especially if you have knee problems.

TAKE CARE
If you have neck problems, ensure that the back of the neck stays long throughout.

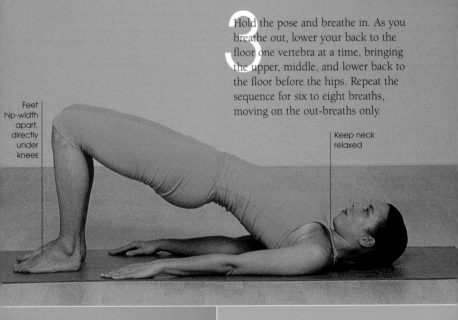

3 Hold the pose and breathe in. As you breathe out, lower your back to the floor one vertebra at a time, bringing the upper, middle, and lower back to the floor before the hips. Repeat the sequence for six to eight breaths, moving on the out-breaths only.

Feet hip-width apart, directly under knees

Keep neck relaxed

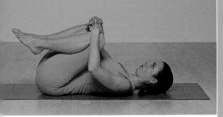

4 When you have completed the practice, draw the knees in towards the chest and wrap the arms around the knees. Relax the shoulders. Rock slowly from side to side and feel your back moving against the floor.

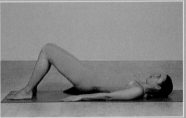

ALTERNATIVE
If you have a back problem, try taking the feet a little further away from the hips when you begin, and lift only the hips off the floor, not the whole back.

legs
up the wall

Inverted postures can be particularly restorative, and you do not need to be able to do a Headstand to reap the benefits of inversion. Try Legs up the Wall first if you are new to inverted postures.

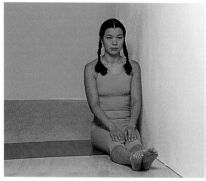 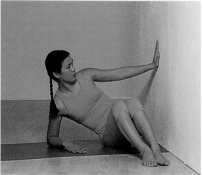

1 Sit up straight with your left hip against a wall. Place your hands on your thighs and breathe easily for a few moments. Draw the knees up.

2 Lean over on to your right elbow and place the left hand against the wall. Swivel your trunk through 90 degrees so that your legs are against the wall and your hips close to the base of it.

TAKE CARE
- If you have HBP, Legs up the Wall is the only suitable inverted posture.
- If you have LBP, come out of any inverted postures really slowly.

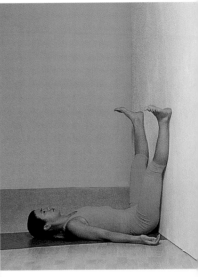

3 Bend your elbows and bring your hands to rest on your stomach. Relax the legs up the wall and stay quietly in this position, observing the flow of the natural breath for two to three minutes.

Keep legs together

Draw chin towards chest to lengthen back of neck

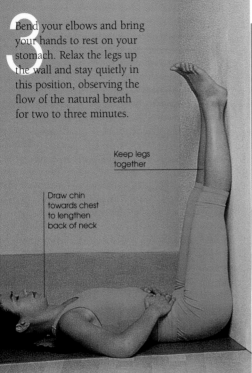

4 Separate the feet, and let your arms rest by your sides, palms up, for a few breaths. To come out of the pose, draw the knees over the chest and roll over to one side. Stay in this position for a few breaths before sitting up. Once sitting, wait for a few breaths before standing up.

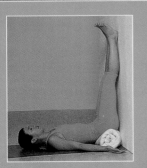

ALTERNATIVE
Place a soft bolster or cushion under the hips if your back is not comfortable when flat on the floor.

half
shoulderstand

This gentle version of Shoulderstand is restorative, quietening the mind while resting the legs and lower body. By using a wall for support, it is easy to learn how to do this inversion.

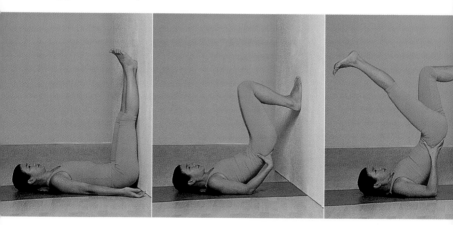

1 Sit with your left hip against a wall. Move into Legs up the Wall (see p.70).

2 Place the feet against the wall and push, raising the hips. Bring the hands to the backs of the hip bones.

3 Lift the heels from the wall and raise the hips higher. Take the right foot off the wall and bring over your head.

TAKE CARE
If you have HBP, a heart condition, detached retina, glaucoma, neck problems, or are overweight, do Legs up the Wall (see p.70).

4 Take the left foot off the wall. Relax the neck and stay for several breaths. Draw the chin gently towards the chest to lengthen the back of the neck. Breathe normally, stretching the soles of the feet towards the ceiling and lengthening through the legs and spine.

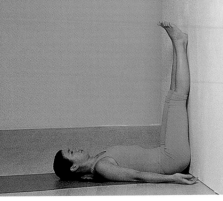

Keep legs
straight and
together

5 Bend your right knee to bring the sole of your right foot back to the wall. Then bring your left foot to the wall. Lower your spine to the floor, keeping the back supported as you come down. Take your arms out to the side.

6 To come out of the pose, draw the knees over the chest and roll on to your right side. Stay with the head down for several breaths. Sit up slowly, particularly if you have LBP.

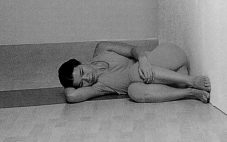

Keep elbows well tucked
in for support

easy fish

This posture opens the hips and shoulders, while supporting the back. Modified Fish provides an excellent counterstretch for the back and the neck after doing the Half Shoulderstand (see p.72).

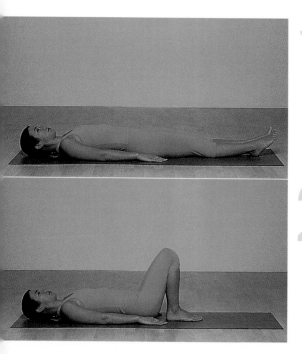

1 Lie on your back with your legs outstretched and your feet hip-width apart. Place your arms by your sides, palms facing downwards. Look up at the ceiling.

2 Draw up the knees and place the soles of your feet flat on the floor close to the hips. Lengthen the back of the neck by drawing the chin down a little towards the chest.

3 Cross your feet at the ankles, and allow the knees to drop out to the sides – right knee to the right side, left knee to the left – so that you are lying in a cross-legged position. Allow the hip joints to relax and open. Do not overarch the back.

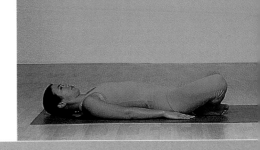

4 Bring your arms up and clasp your hands to cradle the head. Let the elbows sink to the floor. Observe the natural rise and fall of the abdomen with the breath for several breaths. Uncross the ankles, cross them the other way, and stay for several more breaths. To come out of the pose, bring the knees back together and slide the feet away.

Do not force knees to floor

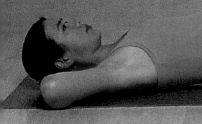

ALTERNATIVE
If you have lower back pain, sacro-iliac problems, or simply stiff hips, support either or both legs by tucking a bolster or cushion under the thighs. Then let the thighs relax down on to the support.

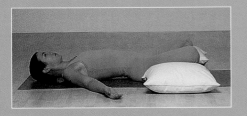

roaring lion

Roaring Lion posture is a great stress reliever. It stretches the face, jaw, and throat, while simultaneously releasing any sense of being under pressure, whether from the demands of work or home.

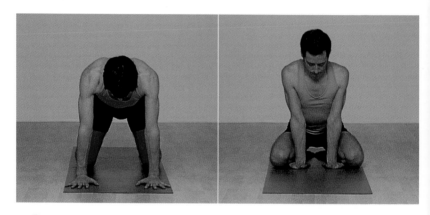

1 Begin on all fours, the hands directly under the shoulders, the feet and knees about hip-width apart. Spread your fingers and look down.

2 Sit back on your heels with the knees wider than the hips and the feet close together. Position the hands on the floor inside the knees, and turn the hands so that the heels of the hands point forwards. Lift the breastbone and look slightly forwards.

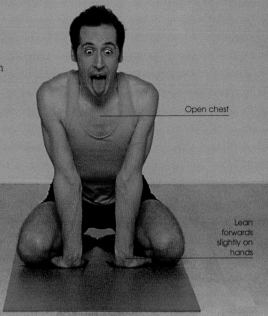

3 Breathe in deeply. As you breathe out, open your mouth wide and stretch the tip of the tongue down to the chin. Open the eyes wide and look up, as you exhale with a soft, continuous "haaaa" sound. The sound should be soft, not harsh or unduly loud, and should last the length of the exhalation. If your throat feels rough afterwards, you are practising too strongly.

Open chest

Lean forwards slightly on hands

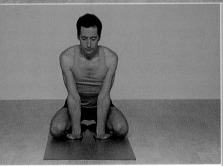

4 As you breathe in, slowly draw in the relaxed tongue, relax the face, and close the mouth. Breathe normally for a few breaths, feeling the effects, then repeat two or three times.

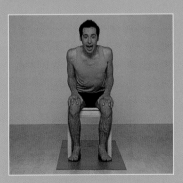

ALTERNATIVE

If you have knee problems or painful wrists, sit on a chair. Lean forwards, the hands placed lightly on the thighs.

cat

Cat is practised slowly, with the movements initiated from the tailbone. It works the back, easing out tension and strengthening the muscles. Learn the positions first, then link them to the breath.

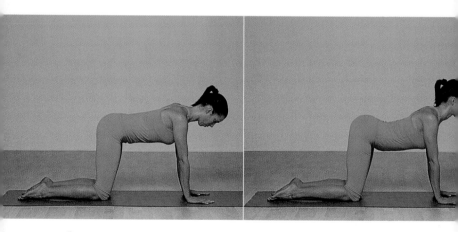

1 Kneel on all fours, hands under the shoulders and knees under the hips. Push the hands into the floor to prevent the shoulders from sagging. Look down at the floor.

2 As you breathe in, begin to lift the tailbone up away from the floor, so that the lower back dips towards the floor. Continue to lift the tailbone and feel first the middle of the back dip, then the upper back. Look at the floor about 1 m (3 ft) in front of you.

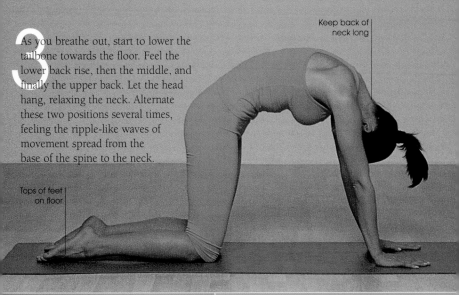

3 As you breathe out, start to lower the tailbone towards the floor. Feel the lower back rise, then the middle, and finally the upper back. Let the head hang, relaxing the neck. Alternate these two positions several times, feeling the ripple-like waves of movement spread from the base of the spine to the neck.

Keep back of neck long

Tops of feet on floor

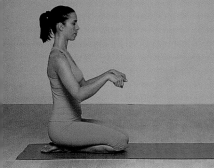

4 On an out-breath, sit back on your heels with your arms in front. Slowly circle the hands at the wrists a few times in each direction to ease them after this weight-bearing posture.

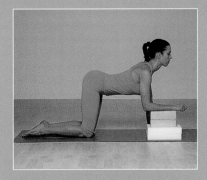

ALTERNATIVE

If one or both your wrists are painful when your hands are bearing your weight or if you have weak wrists, support the body by placing one or both forearms on blocks.

cat
balance

This variation of the Cat pose is unusual in that it stretches the body diagonally. It also encourages balance, and a sense of focus. Keep the spine and pelvis in a neutral position throughout.

1 Kneel on all fours, the knees beneath the hips, the feet and knees a little apart. Look down at the floor. Spread the fingers and hold the neck in line.

2 On an in-breath, lift the left leg and stretch it out behind you. Do not look up as this tightens the neck. Pause for a few breaths to get your balance.

3 On an in-breath, slowly take the right arm out in front, parallel to the floor. Stretch the raised hand and foot away from each other. Breathe easily. Slowly release the pose and repeat, stretching out the right leg and the left arm.

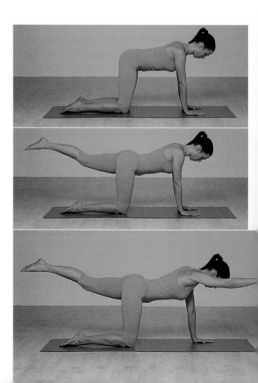

hare

Hare gently stretches the back, hips, knees, and ankles. It is a restorative pose that helps you to develop a deep sense of calm by taking your attention inwards. (For Alternatives, see Child, p.83.)

1 Kneel and sit back on your heels, looking straight ahead. Bring the breastbone up and relax the shoulders. Let your arms hang either side of the body. Lengthen through the spine. Breathe in.

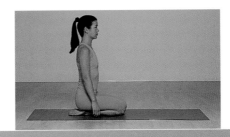

2 As you exhale, fold forwards from the hips, stretching the arms out along the floor in front of you and bringing the forehead to the floor between the arms. Stay for several breaths. To come out of the pose, walk your hands towards your body and sit up on your heels.

If your ankles are uncomfortable, place a folded cloth beneath them for support.

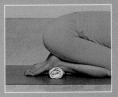

Hands and elbows flat on floor

child

Child is a deeply calming pose that gently stretches the spine and postural muscles in the back, while taking your attention inwards. It is a good posture for developing breath awareness.

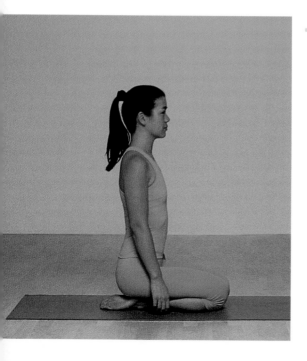

1 Kneel and sit back on your heels. Keep the breastbone up and the shoulders relaxed. Allow your arms to hang down either side of your body. Lengthen through the spine and look straight ahead. Breathe in.

2 As you exhale, fold forward, tucking the chin in to bring the head to the floor. Allow the weight of the arms to draw the shoulders gently towards the floor. Stay for several breaths. To come out of the pose, bring the palms of your hands to the floor and push up slowly..

Feel the stretch across the upper back

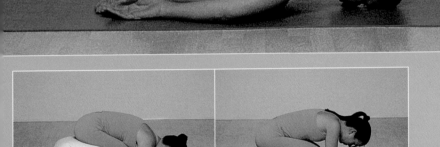

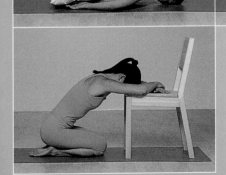

ALTERNATIVES

If your knees are uncomfortable, place a small pillow between the hips and the heels to lift the hips a little. If you find it difficult to bring your head to the floor, rest it on the two fists, one on top of the other. If you have HBP, detached retina, glaucoma or back problems, rest your head on the seat of a chair.

seated forward stretch

This posture has marked quietening effects, and is often used in yoga therapy to reduce stress. It encourages flexibility in the spine and hamstrings, and allows you to focus on inner awareness.

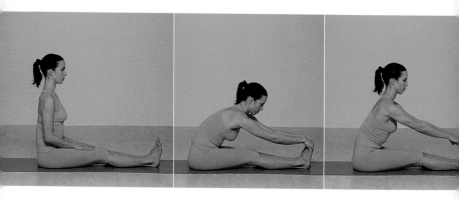

1 Set a firm pillow or bolster close by. Sit with your legs straight out in front of you, feet together. Let your hands rest lightly on your thighs. Look straight ahead and take a few breaths to centre yourself.

2 Breathing out, lift the breastbone and lengthen the spine. Relax the shoulders. Stretch forwards from the hips and hold the toes, ankles, or shins, depending on your level of flexibility.

3 As you breathe in, lift up the breastbone and lengthen the spine, keeping hold of the toes. Keep the legs and arms straight, and look straight ahead.

4 As you breathe out, fold forwards again, bending the elbows and relaxing the neck. Bring your head to your knees, rounding your back. Keep the legs straight. Repeat Steps 3 and 4 for four to six breaths.

Keep neck relaxed

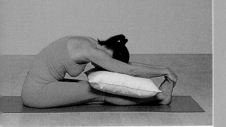

5 Place a firm pillow, bolster, or folded blanket on your legs below your knees. Relax forward over the support and hold for a further four to six breaths. Be aware of the flow of the natural breath.

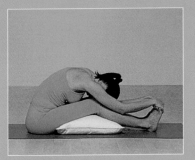

ALTERNATIVE

If you have back problems, a hernia, or tight hamstrings, do not strain to reach toes. Place a cushion under the knees.

cobbler

Cobbler pose opens the hips, while lengthening the spine upwards. Practised with the breath, it is one of the most quietening of all yoga postures, and a wonderful stress reliever.

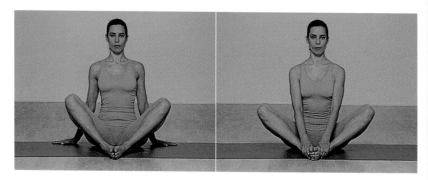

1 Sit with your legs stretched out in front of you. Place your hands on the floor on either side of your body and lean back a little. Bend the knees and swing the soles of your feet together on the floor in front of you.

2 Reach forward and clasp the hands around the feet. Breathing in, sit up straight, lifting the breastbone and lengthening the spine upwards. Look straight ahead.

TAKE CARE
• If your back rounds, sit on a foam block or small cushion.
• If you have stiff hips, place a cushion under each thigh for support.

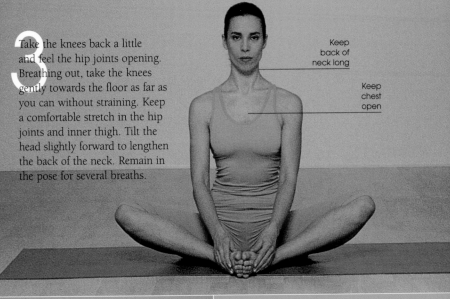

3 Take the knees back a little and feel the hip joints opening. Breathing out, take the knees gently towards the floor as far as you can without straining. Keep a comfortable stretch in the hip joints and inner thigh. Tilt the head slightly forward to lengthen the back of the neck. Remain in the pose for several breaths.

Keep back of neck long

Keep chest open

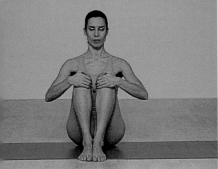

4 To come out of the pose, release the feet and draw the knees together. Place your hands on your knees and roll the legs from side to side several times to ease the hips.

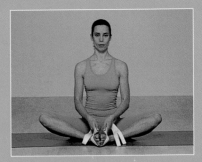

ALTERNATIVE

If you find it difficult to sit up straight while holding on to the feet, use a belt looped around the feet. Hold on to the belt near to the feet, so that the shoulders are gently pulled down.

kneeling
stretch sequence

This is a calming sequence that helps you unwind and balance your energy. It is especially beneficial at the end of a stressful day, when it will refresh your mind and body, enabling you to enjoy the evening.

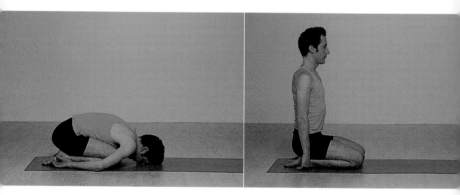

1 Kneel and sit back on your heels, your arms by the sides of your body. As you breathe out, fold forwards into Child (see p.82), bringing the upper body on to the thighs.

2 Breathe in and come back up to sitting on your heels. Let your arms hang down by the sides of your body. Look straight ahead. Breathe out.

TAKE CARE
• Take your time to learn the sequence, matching it to the breathing pattern.
• Practise within your natural breathing capacity, gradually developing slow, rhythmic breathing.

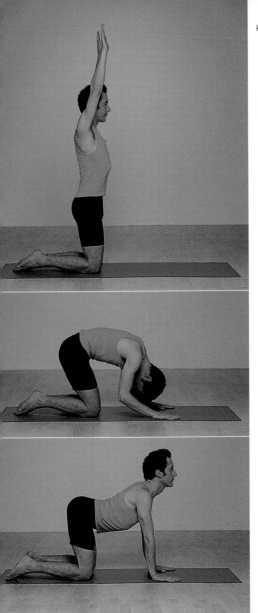

Breathing in, come up on to your knees. At the same time, raise the arms up above the head. Soften the elbows as the arms come up, palms facing forwards, shoulders relaxed. Look straight ahead.

Breathing out, curl the tailbone under and bring the hips down towards the heels, stopping before you reach them. Let the hands come lightly to the floor in front of you and the head hang in a kneeling Forward Bend.

Breathing in, bring the head and chest up, so that you are in an all-fours position. Stretch the breastbone forward and bring the tailbone up, letting the back sink down into the first part of Cat (see p.78). ▶

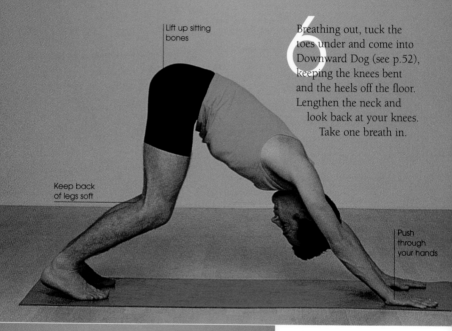

Lift up sitting bones

Keep back of legs soft

6 Breathing out, tuck the toes under and come into Downward Dog (see p.52), keeping the knees bent and the heels off the floor. Lengthen the neck and look back at your knees. Take one breath in.

Push through your hands

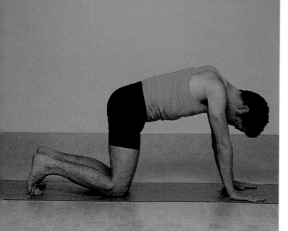

7 Breathing out, come back on to all fours, your knees directly underneath your hips. Look down at the floor. Breathe in.

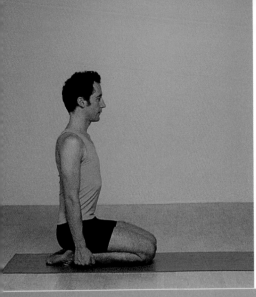

Breathing out, come back up to kneeling, sitting on your heels. Let your arms hang down by your sides. Look straight ahead and take a breath in.

Feel stretch across back

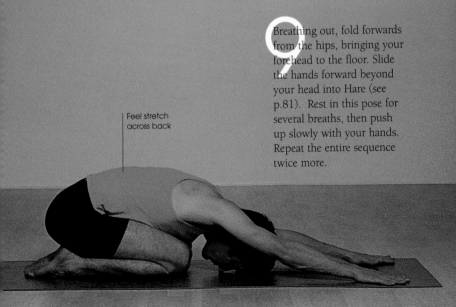

Breathing out, fold forwards from the hips, bringing your forehead to the floor. Slide the hands forward beyond your head into Hare (see p.81). Rest in this pose for several breaths, then push up slowly with your hands. Repeat the entire sequence twice more.

sitting twist

Sitting twists help to maintain flexibility in the back, while easing out muscle tension. This posture is also very stress-relieving as it helps you to connect with your breath at a deep level.

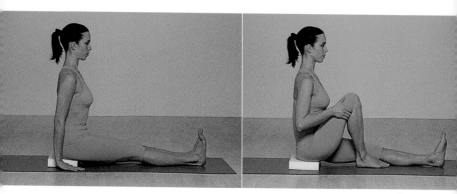

1 Sit on a foam block or small cushion, with the legs straight out in front of you and the feet together. Lift the breastbone and lengthen the spine upwards. Relax the shoulders and look straight ahead.

2 Place your hands under the right knee and draw the knee up. Flex the left foot and stretch the heel of the left leg away from you. Continue to look straight ahead.

TAKE CARE

Twist within comfortable limits. It is important to turn the neck last, avoiding any sense of strain in this area.

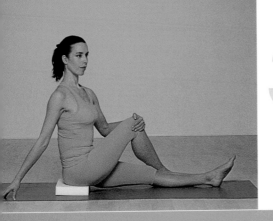

3 Take the right foot across the left leg, setting it down beside the left calf. Clasp both hands over the bent knee and lengthen the spine. Bring the fingers of the right hand to the floor behind you. Breathe in as you lengthen through the upper body.

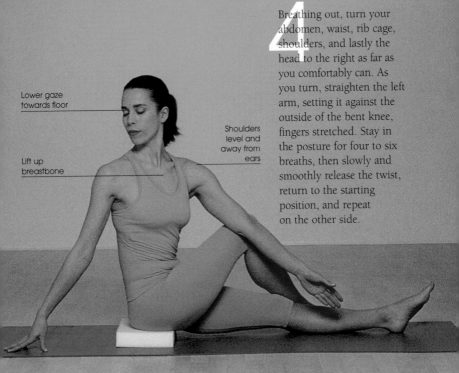

Lower gaze towards floor

Lift up breastbone

Shoulders level and away from ears

4 Breathing out, turn your abdomen, waist, rib cage, shoulders, and lastly the head to the right as far as you comfortably can. As you turn, straighten the left arm, setting it against the outside of the bent knee, fingers stretched. Stay in the posture for four to six breaths, then slowly and smoothly release the twist, return to the starting position, and repeat on the other side.

chair
twist

Tension in the neck, shoulders, and lower back may set in towards the end of the day after spending hours at your desk. Break up the day and release the tension by doing the Chair Twist in your office.

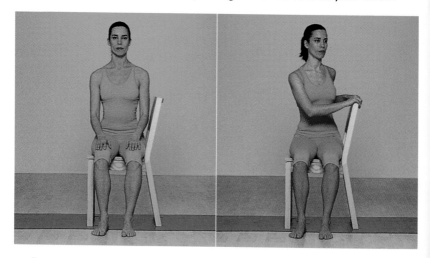

1 Sit sideways on the chair, with your feet on the ground. If the chair is too high, place a telephone directory or similar book under your feet. Place your hands on your thighs and look straight ahead.

2 Lift up the breastbone and take hold of the back of the chair with both hands. Relax the shoulders. Look down slightly. Breathing out, begin to turn the upper body towards the back of the chair, starting with the stomach.

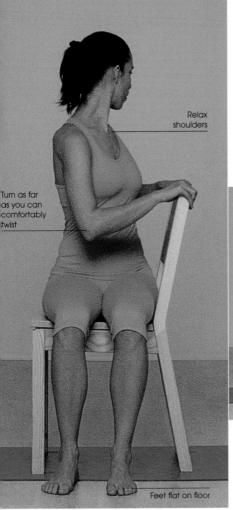

Relax
shoulders

Turn as far
as you can
comfortably
twist

Feet flat on floor

3 Still breathing out, turn the waist, rib cage, and shoulders, keeping the breastbone up and shoulders relaxed. Finally, turn the head as far as it will comfortably go. Relax the face and connect with the breath for several breaths.

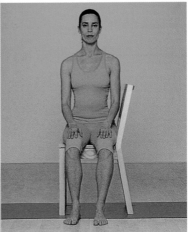

4 On an out-breath, slowly release the pose and come back to the starting position. Swivel around on the chair to face the opposite direction and practise the posture on the other side.

TAKE CARE
Turn each part of the trunk only to your maximum comfortable limit: there should be no strain at any time.

breathing
practices & mudras

Breathing practices improve your awareness of the breath, and are particularly useful in quietening the mind for meditation. Mudras are traditional hand gestures that help you to centre yourself.

The breathing practices described on these four pages will help improve your breath awareness and encourage calmness and mental clarity. They are generally practised after doing some yoga postures, or some simple stretching. Physical movement helps loosen up the body, so that it is easier for you to be relaxed during the breathing practices. You might like to use a mudra in conjunction with a breathing practice to improve its effectiveness.

Audible breath

A simple but effective breathing practice to begin with is known as audible breath. This practice helps to make the breath smooth and even, calms and centres the mind, and is

a proven stress reliever. It can also be used during posture work to help you to remain focused.

Begin with the preliminary practice described below. When you have got a feel for this, try to achieve

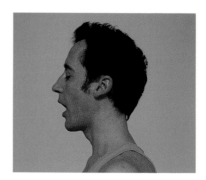

Breathe through the mouth. Slightly close the throat and make a sighing "Ahhhh" sound as you breathe in and a sighing "Haaa" sound as you breathe out.

the same sound in the throat while breathing with your mouth closed. It helps to think that you are breathing through a hole in the front of the throat. Breathe smoothly and evenly, and keep your awareness on the breath. The sound of the breath can be quite subtle; only you need hear it.

Using mudras

There are many mudras, or hand gestures, used in yoga practice. The centring mudra shown on this page (see right) helps you to quieten quickly when you are feeling stressed. This enables you to break the stress cycle effortlessly, making you feel much calmer within minutes. Practising this mudra also acts to remind you of the link between the individual and universal consciousness – that we are all interconnected, never unsupported.

The centring mudra can be very helpful at any time of the day, whatever your situation. It can be used in an unobtrusive way at work, socially, and at times of stress, with the hands in any convenient position – they do not have to be supported.

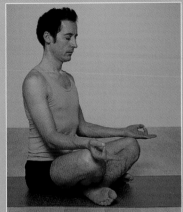

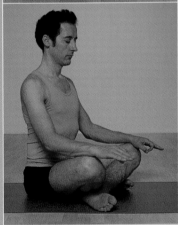

MUDRA FOR CENTRING

Bring the tip of each index finger and thumb together lightly. Rest the hands on the thighs or the knees. During the daytime have the palms facing upwards, and after dark have the palms facing downwards.

alternate nostril breathing

Breathing through alternate nostrils has a balancing effect on the mind, body, and emotions. As you practise the breathing, let go of any tension in the body. If you are left-handed, adapt the instructions below to suit. Do several rounds. When you are comfortable with the practice, begin to lengthen the out-breath until it is twice as long as the in-breath.

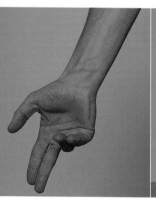 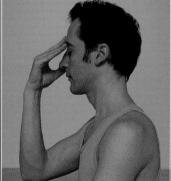 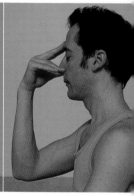

1 Sit cross-legged on the floor. Lift the breastbone and relax the shoulders. Take your right hand and separate the index and middle fingers from the thumb and the ring and little finger. Place the index and middle fingers in the centre of the forehead.

2 Connect with your natural breath. Close the right nostril with your thumb and breathe in through the left nostril.

3 Close the left nostril with your ring and little finger and open the right. Breathe out through the right, then breathe back in through the right. Close the right nostril, open the left, and breathe out through that. This completes one round.

sounds breathing

This practice uses the vibrational power of sound to relax the body and mind, and helps to make the breath smooth and even. Once you are familiar with the practice you can do it without making a sound. Inhale, and, as you exhale soundlessly, simply visualize the "ahhhh", "ohhhh", and "mmmm" sounds for the length of each out-breath.

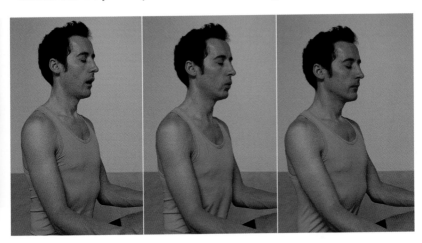

1 Sit cross-legged and close your eyes. Lift the breastbone and relax the shoulders. Inhale and, as you breathe out, make the sound "ahhhh". Feel the vibrations in the abdomen. Repeat twice more.

2 Breathe in and, as you breathe out, make the sound "ohhhh" for the length of the out-breath. This time feel the vibrations in the chest. Repeat this sound twice more.

3 For the length of the next out-breath, make the sound "mmmm". As you do so, feel the vibrations in the throat and the head. Repeat this sound twice more. Be aware of the stillness within, then open your eyes.

meditation

Meditation is a practice that allows the mind to quieten, giving a lasting sense of inner peace and harmony. It helps to keep your mind clear throughout the day and can aid sleep at night.

Sit in a comfortable but alert way, either cross-legged on the floor (using a block, cushion, or blanket if you prefer) or upright in a chair. Bring the index finger and thumb of each hand together and rest the hands on your knees or thighs. This is the mudra that allows you to centre yourself more effectively and connects you to the universal consciousness (see p.97).

PRACTICAL MATTERS

• Choose a posture that you will be able to sustain easily for some time; for example, sitting cross-legged, kneeling, or sitting upright on a chair.
• Make sure that the temperature of the room is comfortable. You may need to put on some warmer clothes if you have been doing posture work.

Scan the body, letting go of any tension you are holding (in your face, neck, shoulders, upper body, hips, legs, and feet). Close your eyes and let your breath settle into an easy, regular rhythm. Do not try actively to shut out any noises or other sensations. Allow them to exist and withdraw your senses from them as you focus on your breath. Be aware of the coolness of the air in the openings of the nostrils as you breathe in and the warmth of the air there as you breathe out.

To begin with, thoughts will inevitably arise and sensations will distract you. You cannot force the mind to be empty. But do not let yourself react to these disturbances.

Observe them objectively as they come into the mind and let them go as you continue to focus on the breath. Do not let yourself be carried away on a train of thought.

Using visualization

Bring your awareness to your natural breath. As you draw the breath in, visualize the breath entering your body through the base of your spine and moving gently up the spine until it fills your lungs. As you breathe out, visualize the breath flowing back down the spine and leaving the body.

Visualize the breath as a fine mist or as a soft white light. Alternatively, if you find visualization difficult, simply focus on the sense of movement as the breath passes up and down the spine. You may like to say to yourself "up" as you breathe in, and "down" as you breathe out.

Allow the practice to be easy, without any sense of strain. If you notice that your mind has wandered, gently bring it back to "seeing" the flow of the breath up and down the spine. After two to three minutes you

will notice that you are feeling quietly energized and calmer than before.

Practise this visualization meditation for up to 10 minutes, then open your eyes. Once you are accustomed to the practice, you will be able to use it in any situation and posture – sitting or standing, eyes open or closed, and the hands relaxed in any comfortable position.

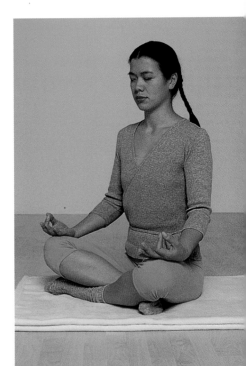

relaxation

Stress affects the mind and the body equally. It can be difficult for a busy mind to quieten directly, but when you learn to relax the body, you will find that your mind soon settles and becomes calm.

Relaxation is a skill that improves with regular practice, as the body and mind become accustomed to releasing tension.

There are two relaxation practices described on the next four pages. The instant relaxation practice can be used at any time of the day or night, anywhere, sitting or standing. For the 10-minute relaxation practice, you will need to lie down in a place where you are guaranteed privacy and quiet for at least 10 minutes. It provides a deep relaxation and is ideal when you have plenty of time.

Relaxation benefits

Use the instant relaxation technique (see opposite) whenever you feel stress building up during the day.

Once you have learned this simple and unobtrusive practice, you will also find it extremely useful to try in specific situations, for example, just before a high-pressure meeting, interview, or presentation.

Ten minutes or so lying down in deep relaxation allows you to recharge your batteries and let go of any feeling of being under pressure. Many people find it especially beneficial to practise deep relaxation at the end of their yoga session, to reinforce the restorative and regenerative benefits. Try to make sure that you will not be disturbed. Loosen any tight clothing and wear a jumper or cover yourself with a blanket: the body loses heat as the blood vessels in the skin relax.

instant relaxation

It is invaluable to be able to relax at any time, in any situation. Using this simple technique, you will quickly learn to be composed and stress-free, no matter what is going on around you. Repeat this instant relaxation practice as soon as you begin to feel any tension building up again.

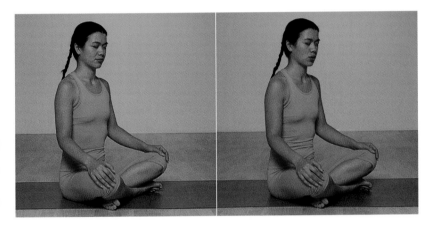

1 Sit cross-legged on the floor, your hands resting on your knees. Close your eyes. Turn your attention inwards and become aware of the flow of the natural breath. Breathe in through the nose as you take your awareness to your jaw.

2 Breathe out in an even stream through slightly pursed lips, softly "blowing the breath away" and with it the stress in your jaw. With the next breath in, be aware of the shoulders, and then blow out the tension with the out-breath. On the next in-breath focus on the hands. As you breathe out, let them become passive. Move your awareness between these areas for several breaths, keeping each one relaxed and soft.

10-minute relaxation

Try recording this guided relaxation, or ask a friend to read it to you slowly. This allows you to relax to the deepest level. Lie on your back with your legs outstretched, feet more than hip-width apart. Let the feet roll out. (If you have lower back problems, keep your knees bent.) Ease the shoulders down to the floor. Take the arms away from the body and turn the inner elbows and palms up to the ceiling. Lengthen the back of the neck, bringing the chin towards the chest. Close the eyes. Allow the body to become still.

Scanning the body

Take your awareness around each part of the right side of the body. Be aware of the thumb, fingers, palm of right hand, back of hand, wrist, lower arm, elbow, upper arm, shoulder, armpit, right side of chest, right side of waist, right hip, right thigh, kneecap, back of knee, shin, calf muscle, ankle, heel, sole of foot, top of foot, toes.

Now take your attention to the left side of the body. Be aware of the thumb, fingers, palm of the left hand, back of hand, wrist. Be aware of the lower arm, elbow, upper arm, shoulder, armpit, left side of chest, left side of waist, left hip. Now be aware of the left thigh, kneecap, back of knee, shin, calf muscle, ankle, heel, sole of foot, top of foot, toes.

Take your awareness to the back of the body. Be aware of the back of the head, back of the neck, backs of shoulders, left shoulder blade, right shoulder blade, middle of back, lower back, left buttock, right buttock, back of left thigh, back of right thigh, back of left knee, back of right knee, left calf, right calf, left heel, right heel, sole of left foot, sole of right foot.

Take your attention to the top of your head. Now to the front of the body. Be aware of the forehead, left eyebrow, right eyebrow, space between eyebrows, left eyelid, right eyelid, left eyeball, right eyeball. Be aware of the bridge of the nose, left nostril, right nostril, left cheekbone, right cheekbone, upper lip, inside the mouth – teeth, gums, tongue – the lower lip, chin, under the chin, front of throat, left side of neck, right side of neck, left collarbone, right collarbone, left side of chest, right side of chest, front of chest, abdomen. Now be aware of the whole body.

Focusing inwards

Turn your attention inwards and feel how tranquil your body has become. Become aware of the quietness of your breath, which does not disturb the stillness of your body as it flows gently in and out. Stay with your breath for a little while and, as you do, experience the sense of inner quietness, inner peace – feel connected with your inner self at the deepest level. Stay in this relaxing posture for two to 10 minutes.

Coming out

When you are ready, draw your awareness outwards again. Be aware of the floor beneath you, the room around you, the sounds that you can hear. Begin to breathe a little more deeply, then start slowly to move the fingers and toes, ankles, arms, and legs. Shrug the shoulders, move the neck, face, and scalp. Take the arms back behind the head and stretch out the body right to the fingertips and down to the heels and toes. Now draw the knees over the chest, wrap the arms around the knees, relax the shoulders, and rock slowly from side to side, feeling your back move against the floor. Now roll over to the right and sit up slowly.

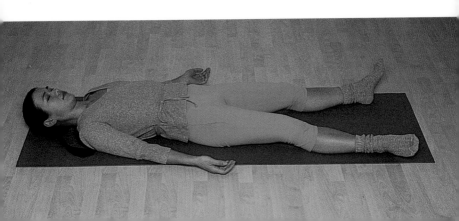

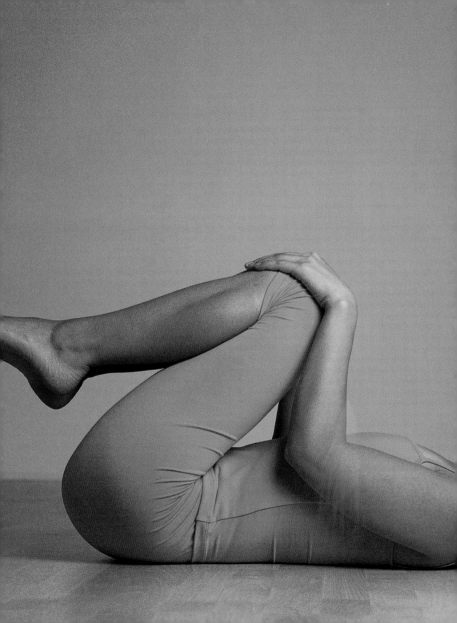

programmes

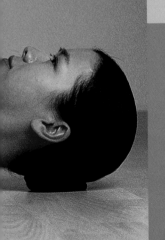

Here are eight programmes for those times in the day when you need to de-stress. Remember to take time to centre yourself before doing them and time to absorb their effects afterwards. Their benefits will be greatly enhanced if you remember that yoga is also about lifestyle and attitude.

1 preparing
for the day

Early morning is the traditional time for yoga practice. Take a few moments to become centred first. This will enable you to develop a sense of calm that will help see you through any stresses in the day ahead. You may feel stiff after sleep, so work gently to open up tight areas, letting your energy flow easily around the body.

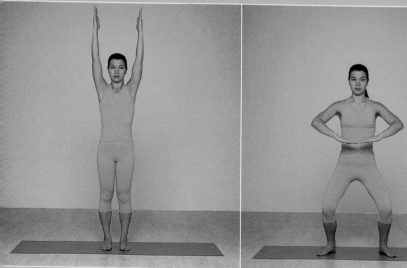

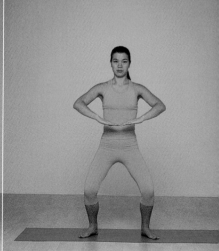

1 Standing Upward Stretch (see p.34)

2 Cafetière Stretch (see p.31)

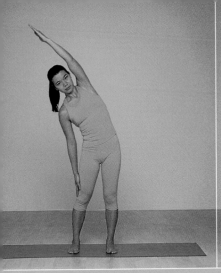

3 Standing Side Stretch (see p.37)

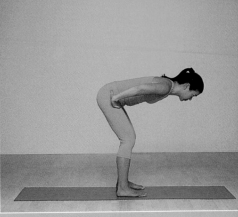

4 Half Forward Bend (see p.35)

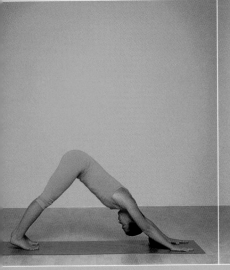

5 Downward Dog (see pp.52–53)

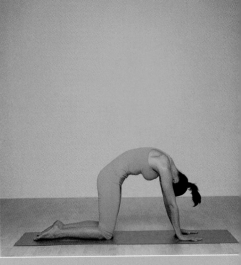

6 Cat (see pp.78–79)

2 work-time stretch

Working indoors in an office environment can make you feel in need of a good stretch. This programme does not require you to get down on the floor; you can stand or sit on an upright chair. The postures may be used together during a short break, but are equally effective practised separately at intervals during your working hours.

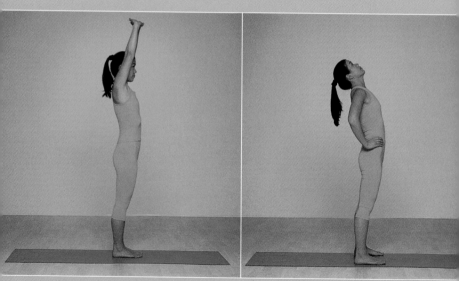

1 **Standing Arm Stretches** (see p.30)

2 **Standing Back Arch** (see p.36)

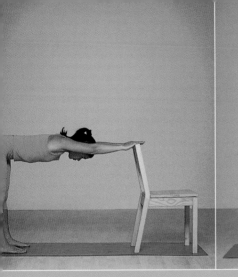

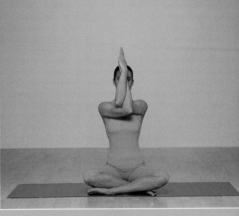

③ Forward Bend using a Chair (see p.45)

④ Eagle (see pp.40–41)

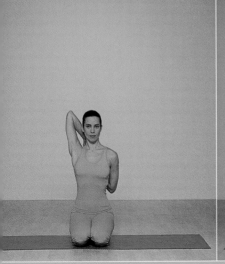

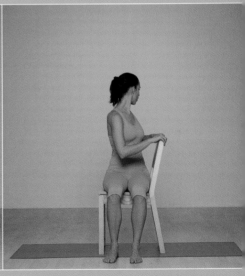

⑤ Cow (see pp.42–43)

⑥ Chair Twist (see pp.94–95)

3 courage
booster

Challenging situations at work sometimes cause stress levels to rocket. An important interview or giving a presentation can deplete your reserves, leaving you exhausted. This programme will boost your energy and build confidence, so that you appear calm and perform well when it counts. Try to find somewhere quiet to practise.

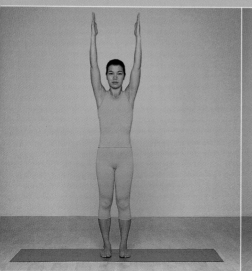

1 Standing Upward Stretch (see p.34)

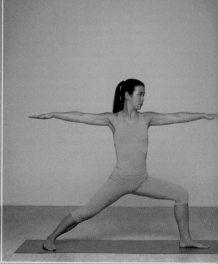

2 Side Warrior (see pp.48–49)

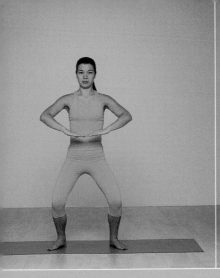

3 Cafetière Stretch (see p.31)

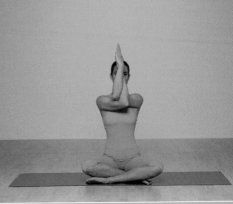

4 Eagle (see pp.40–41)

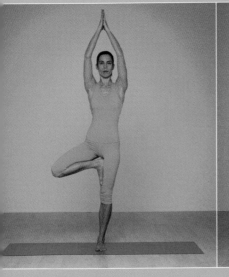

5 Tree (see pp.46–47)

6 Roaring Lion (see pp.76–77)

4 survival tactics

Sometimes it all gets too much – something triggers a sudden increase in your stress levels. This programme is designed for such emergencies! These practices use your breath to enable you to become focused and centred, so that you relax and regain your poise. Memorize the sequence, ready to recall when the need arises.

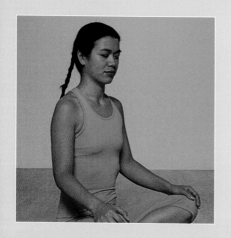

1 Instant Relaxation (see p.103)

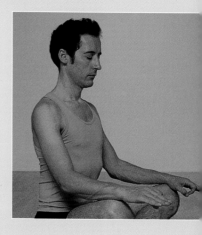

2 Centring Mudra (see p.97)

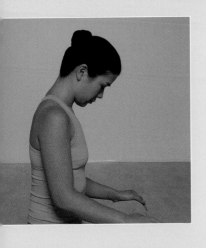

3 Neck Stretches (see pp.32–33)

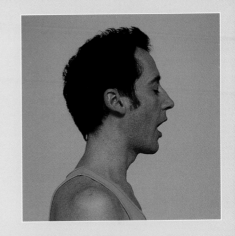

4 Audible Breath (see p.96)

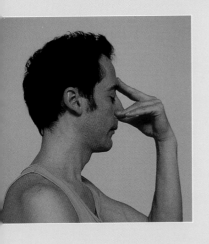

5 Alternate Nostril Breathing (see p.98)

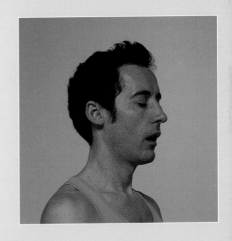

6 Sounds Breathing (see p.99)

5 after-work energizer

After work can sometimes be the only time you have to socialize with your friends; however, by the end of the day, it can be hard to find the energy to enjoy yourself. This programme is designed to help you to let go of work problems, create some vitality, and still have enough time to freshen up before you leave the office!

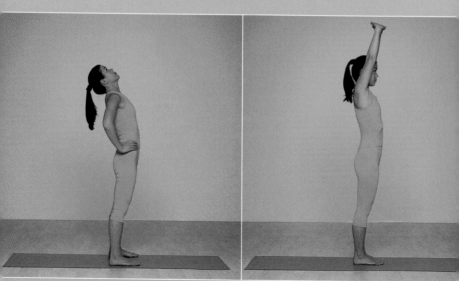

❶ Standing Back Arch (see p.36)

❷ Standing Arm Stretches (see p.30)

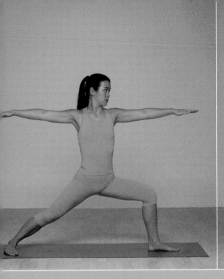

3 Side Warrior (see pp.48–49)

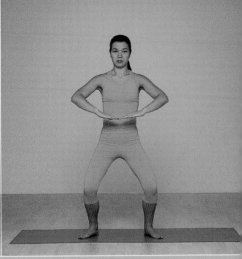

4 Cafetière Stretch (see p.31)

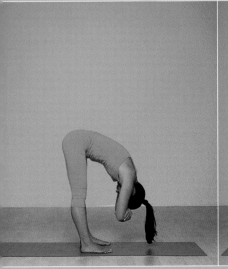

5 Forward Bend (see pp.44–45)

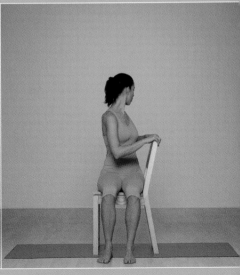

6 Chair Twist (see pp.94–95)

6 evening
pick-me-up

This programme can be used to prepare you for the evening ahead when you have access to floor space and comfortable clothing. Back-arching postures release stress and raise your energy levels, helping you to let go of the work of the day; the simple inversion restores your sense of inner calm while resting the legs.

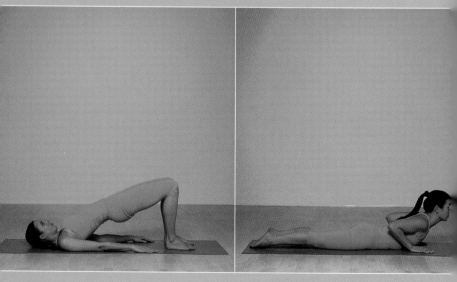

1 Bridge (see pp.68–69)

2 Cobra (see pp.54–55)

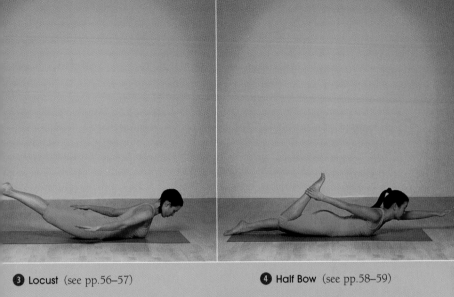

3 Locust (see pp.56–57)

4 Half Bow (see pp.58–59)

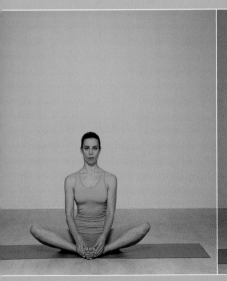

5 Cobbler (see pp.86–87)

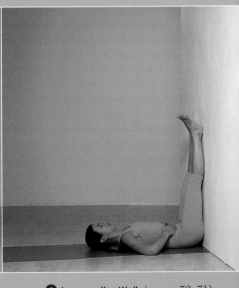

6 Legs up the Wall (see pp.70–71)

7 evening
relaxer

If you are not going out for the evening, do this gentle, slow yoga practice at home, which will help you to unwind and cast off all the accumulated stress of the day. These postures, practised in harmony with the breath, are time-honoured ways of relieving physical tension and releasing feelings of being under pressure.

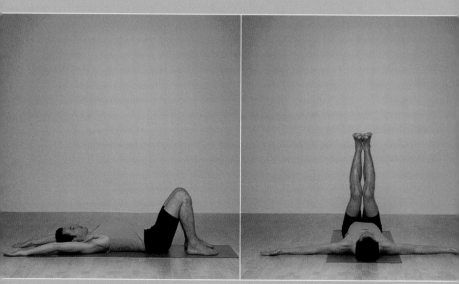

1 Supine Arms Over Head (see p.26)

2 Supine Legs Up Arms Out (see p.2

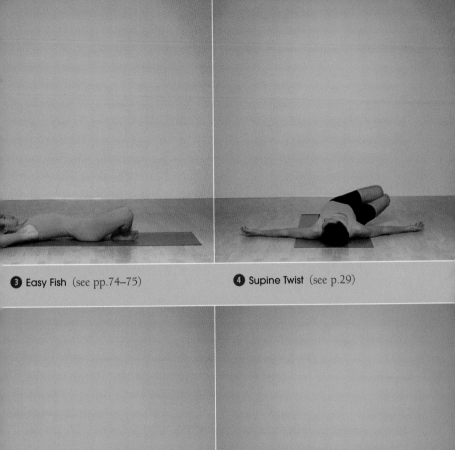

3 Easy Fish (see pp.74–75)

4 Supine Twist (see p.29)

5 Cat (see pp.78–79)

6 Seated Forward Stretch (see pp.84–85)

8 weekend invigorator

Always try to build in some regular yoga time at the weekend. This programme provides a longer practice, incorporating a balanced series of postures to open and stretch every part of your body. As you practise, you will feel your energy flowing more freely, while your sense of general well-being is enhanced and the mind calmed.

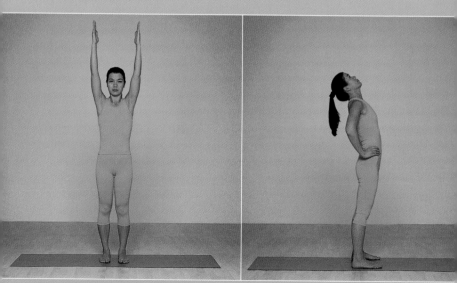

1 **Standing Upward Stretch** (see p.34)

2 **Standing Back Arch** (see p.36)

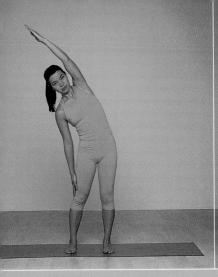

3 Standing Side Stretch (see p.37)

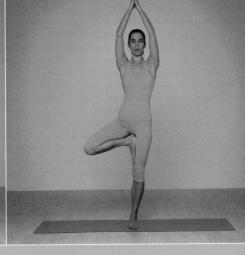

4 Lunge Warrior (see pp.50–51)

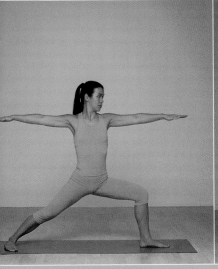

5 Side Warrior (see pp.48–49)

6 Tree (see pp.46–47) ▶

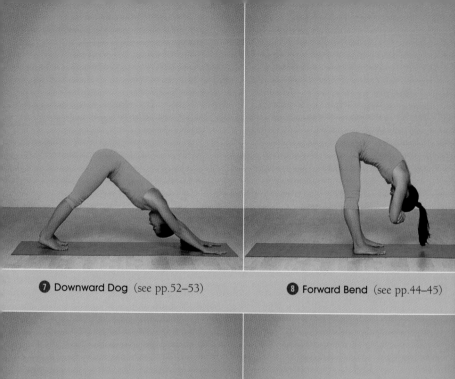

7 Downward Dog (see pp.52–53)

8 Forward Bend (see pp.44–45)

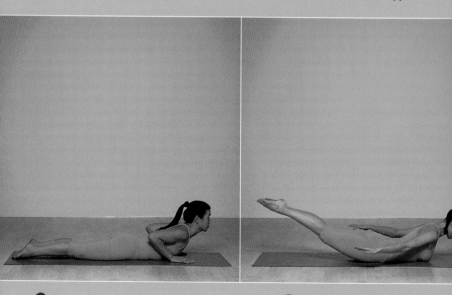

9 Cobra (see pp.54–55)

10 Locust (see pp.56–57)

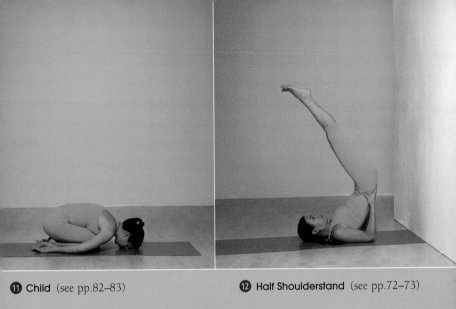

11 Child (see pp.82–83)

12 Half Shoulderstand (see pp.72–73)

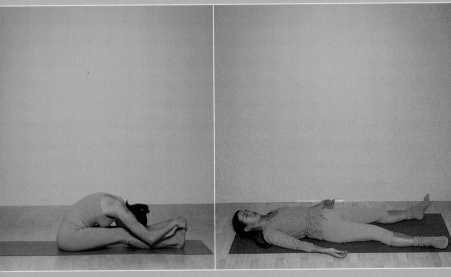

13 Seated Forward Stretch (see pp.84–85)

14 10-Minute Relaxation (see pp.104–105)

Index

Useful organizations

THE BRITISH WHEEL OF YOGA
Tel: 01529 306851;
Website: www.bwy.org.uk
*Provides information on classes, yoga
organizations, and events in the UK.*

www.yogasite.com
*A general source of information on yoga,
with good links, and a teachers' directory
covering the United States, Canada,
Australia, and other countries.*

THE YOGA THERAPY CENTRE
Tel: 020 7869 3040;
Website: www.yogatherapy.org
*The Yoga Biomedical Trust's centre
for yoga therapy, general yoga
classes, workshops and training.*

www.yogafinder.com
*A directory listing yoga teachers,
organizations, and events in the
United States and other countries.*

Acknowledgments

AUTHOR'S ACKNOWLEDGMENTS
I wish to thank Dr Robin Monro of the
Yoga Biomedical Trust for inviting me to
write this book, Peter Falloon-Goodhew
for co-ordinating the project, my family for
their patience, and all who, wittingly and
unwittingly, have shown me the yogic path.

PUBLISHER'S ACKNOWLEDGMENTS
Thanks to Catherine MacKenzie for design
assistance; Helen Ridge, Jane Simmonds,
and Angela Wilkes for editorial assistance;
Dorothy Frame for indexing; Katy Wall for
jacket design; and Anna Bedewell for
additional picture research.

Models: Lee Hamblin, Jane Kemlo,
Jade Littler
Photographer's Assistant: Nick Rayment
Hair and Make-up: Hitoko Honbu
(represented by Hers)
Studio: Air Studios Ltd
Yoga mats: Hugger Mugger Yoga Products,
12 Roseneath Place, Edinburgh EH9 1JB.

Tel: 44 (0) 131 221 9977; **Fax**: 44 (0) 131
2291 9112; **Website**: www.yoga.co.uk;
email: info @huggermugger.co.uk
*In the US, these mats can be obtained
from:* Hugger Mugger Products,
3937 SO 500 W, Salt Lake City, Utah 84123.
Tel: 800 473 4888; **Fax**: 801 268 2629;
Website: www.huggermugger.com
Yoga props: Yoga Matters, 42 Priory Road,
London N8 7EX. Tel: 44 (0) 20 8348 1203;
Website: www.yogamatters.co.uk;
email: enquiries@yogamatters.co.uk